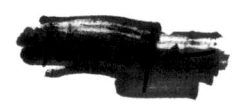

I am so grateful for the initial conversation we had! Thank you so much for sharing your wisdom and experience with me. May God continue to bless you tremendously! Enjoy the book and Soli Deo Gloria!

—Candice

1-27-21

A Quest for Transformation
Getting the Most from This Book

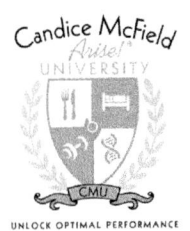

Give a man a fish and he will eat for a day. Teach a man to fish and he will eat for life. CMF teaches fundamentals, hence, clients *Arise!*® and are fit for life!

You will hear many people in fitness state that body transformation relies 80% on diet and 20% on exercise. I completely disagree. Both are equally and independently important. This is why I developed Candice McField University - to help clients *Arise!*® and unlock their optimal performance. Exercise, nutrition, rest, and an understanding of your genetics are all 100% necessary. **Without all four, reaching the upper limits of performance and body transformation is nearly impossible.** The intersection of all four is the bullseye to unleashing full fitness potential. **When you know what to do and understand why you should do it, you are more likely to make wellness a valued part of your lifestyle.**

This book has 21 chapters. Each chapter includes a spiritual lesson, a physical lesson, and corresponding challenges. I strongly recommend you read one chapter per day and act each day of this life-changing quest. Prepare yourself; the next 21 days, will transform *your* life! You will *Arise!*® to a new you!

As for Me and My Body is:
- For males and females of all fitness levels looking to enhance their lives physically, mentally, emotionally, and spiritually
- For people who constantly manage their time
- A 21-day life changing quest in which you will have the opportunity to evaluate, improve, and act in major areas of your life
- Useless without action on your part. It requires you to make sacrifices, commit to obtaining your goals, practice patience, be persistent, exercise discipline, and work hard, and,
- For people of all faiths although there are dominant Christian undertones and themes denoted throughout the book

As for Me and My Body is not:
- Another quick weight loss gimmick or low-quality, falsely advertised product in the multi billion-dollar diet and fitness industry
- For those looking to lose an unhealthy amount of weight in an unrealistic amount of time (long-term healthy weight loss is 1-2 pounds per week)
- Your end-all exhaustive health and fitness solution, you need more than 21 days for that
- In 21 days, you will discover fundamental principles to get you headed in the right direction, and/or propel you to another level regardless of where you begin

In 21 days, you will discover fundamental principles to get you headed in the right direction, and/or propel you to another level regardless of where you begin.

Four Features to Help You
There is a section called, "Unlocking My Optimal Performance" at the end of both the spiritual and physical sections for each day. There you will find:
- **A Moment of Truth.** This is an educational principle that summarizes the day's main learning point. Reflect on this principle throughout the day.

Introduction

- **A Verse/Quote to Remember.** This is a key Bible verse or quote that correlates with the Moment of Truth.
- **A Spiritual Challenge to Accept and Implement.** These challenges are designed to strengthen your relationship with Christ.
- **A Physical Challenge to Accept and Implement.** These challenges are designed to enhance your overall wellness.

My Prayer
I pray God allows me to impact and shape lives - yours included, for years to come. Upon completion of this 21-day life changing quest, I hope you will have strengthened your relationship with Christ by making parallel connections between your spiritual and physical health. I pray your life transforms with increased joy, happiness, energy, and hope. I pray you know that you can conquer all of the health and fitness goals you set for yourself.

Lastly, I pray and encourage you to read, reflect, and implement all 21 principles and challenges without skipping a day. As I mentioned previously, this will take dedication and sacrifice on your part. Schedule your daily reading time and commit. A transformed life awaits you. There is strength in numbers and accountability. There is also something significant about signing your name to a commitment. If you are ready to commit to this, let us sign the pledge together. Are you ready? It is go time!

My Pledge

I, _____ on _____ ,
(Your Name) (Date)

commit to completing the *As for Me and My Body*, 21-Day Quest. I will:

- give my all by implementing any lifestyle changes and sacrifices I may need to make.
- have and keep an open mind to any new paradigms I learn.
- search my heart for inner motivation when I have the desire to backslide to old nutritional, exercise, or sleep habits, or even when I feel like skipping a workout.
- ask _____ to hold me accountable to the goals I set by reporting and sharing with them my triumphs and challenges on a weekly basis.

Complete the following statement:

As for Me and My Body, I will _____

_____

_____

_____   Candice McField
(Your Signature)

Week 1

Day 1

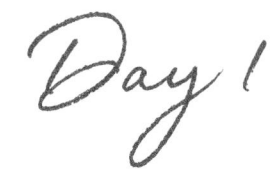

Fitness is a State of Mind

Someone once told me, "God opens doors to create opportunities. Our job is to be obedient, since He controls the outcomes as He plans." Proverbs 19:21 explains this principle. It reads, *"You can make many plans, but the Lord's purpose will prevail."*

I am thankful to have written, *As for Me and My Body*, for any future doors that may open, and for the opportunity to personally connect with you by educating, motivating, and challenging you to reach personal new levels regarding your health. I wrote the word personal because for each of us, our goals are individual. For example, you may want to begin training for a triathlon while someone else may want to commit to eating breakfast daily. We are all at different points but, the great news about being healthy is that the only person in your race is yourself. It is all about you making personal strides and moving forward one small step at a time. This is what makes my heart skip a beat helping you take these steps, hearing your stories, and propelling you through static points.

As this is Day 1, I feel inspired to encourage you to live your dream(s) and to take that leap of faith. Before I begin coaching clients, we speak in depth about their goals and limiting factors. I do this because it is critical for you to have inner motivation. Otherwise, you will not have the inner drive to move through temporary roadblocks during times you find your progress slows or becomes stagnant. Similarly, before I begin to educate you on a variety of health and wellness topics in this book, I challenge you to accept Paul's call to action in Romans 12:1-2 which states,

> "Therefore, I urge you, brothers and sisters, in view of God's mercy, to offer your bodies as a living sacrifice, holy and pleasing to God-this is your true and proper worship. Do not conform to the pattern of this world, but be transformed by the renewing of your mind. Then you will be able to test and approve what God's will is-his good, pleasing and perfect will."

Day 1
Unlocking My Optimal Performance

Moment of Truth: God opens doors to create opportunities. Our job is to be obedient since He controls the outcomes as He plans.

Verse to Remember: "Do not conform to the pattern of this world, but be transformed by the renewing of your mind. Then you will be able to test and approve what God's will is - his good, pleasing and perfect will." Romans 12:2 (NIV)

Challenge to Implement: How have the patterns and comforts of this world, prevented you from walking through a door God has opened for you? In what area of your life do you need to take a leap of faith?

Soli Deo Gloria and Arise!®

Candice

Day 1 - Fitness is a State of Mind

CONGRATULATIONS! You did it! You made the decision to regain control of your overall health and well being through exercise, nutrition, and rest. Great! Before beginning, here is some valuable information.

1. Commitment, consistency, and candor are required.
2. Your efforts determine your results. Do your best for you!
3. This quest goes beyond the physical. Dig deep and renew your thinking.

Whatever your reasons for deciding to improve your fitness, the first step of your journey takes place in your mind.

Fitness is not one dimensional. Physical fitness is just one aspect of the wellness wheel and what goes on in your mind and body is equally important. Fitness requires more than physical strength and endurance; it demands mental focus and proper tools such as good nutrition and patience. Because our physical appearance can significantly impact our mental state, it is important to take stock of where we are, currently.

I encourage you to assess yours as it relates to your desire to dive into a new exercise program. If you are not certain where to begin, try answering these questions.

1. **Are you mentally prepared to begin a fitness program?** It is important to understand your fitness journey is a marathon, not a sprint. There will be triumphs (weight loss, improved mood, etc.), obstacles (e.g., temptation, breaking old habits) and occasionally, setbacks (e.g.,

plateaus).

2. **How much time/effort are you willing to commit to your fitness program?** It takes more than intention to succeed, action is required. Are you willing to make time to set yourself up for success?

As you sit with these questions, be honest with yourself. When you decide that you are all in, consult with your physician before beginning an exercise routine to determine your physical readiness. Do not be discouraged if you must begin slowly. Starting is always better than standing still. Here is to your health!

Day 1 - Fitness is a State of Mind

Day 1
Unlocking My Optimal Performance

Moment of Truth: Whatever your reasons for deciding to improve your fitness, the first step of your journey takes place in your mind.

Quote to Remember: "The health and fitness quest goes beyond the physical. Dig deep and renew your thinking."
~Collier Lunn

Challenge to Implement: Reflect on your reasons for pursuing fitness. List your top three reasons for change below, and use numbers 1-3 to rank them in priority order (#1 being the top reason). Be honest with yourself as your reasons will directly propel your inner motivation. No reason is too small or too grand, and you may have reasons that overlap. Secondly, complete and score the Readiness for Change Questionnaire.

Soli Deo Gloria and Arise!®

Candice

My Reason for Change	Rank

Transformation Readiness Questionnaire

The Transformation Readiness Questionnaire is designed to help you make an honest assessment of your willingness and ability to do the work required to improve your overall physical health.

Often, people think that the desire to make changes is all they need. But desire is not enough. In order to make lasting, positive change, one must be willing and able to implement new behaviors.

One note: Be honest. The purpose of this questionnaire is not to criticize you for your thoughts or actions in the past, rather to discover those areas where you are and/or may not be quite ready to experience transformation.

Questions	Response and Scoring
1. When you look at yourself in the mirror, do you feel embarrassed, unhappy, frustrated, or any other negative emotions?	O Yes, I often feel negative emotions when I look at myself in the mirror. (+3) O I am not sure, as I never really thought about it. (0) O No. For the most part I am happy with the way I look. (-3)
2. Despite any habits or actions of the past, are you willing to accept responsibility for the current condition of your body?	O Yes, I am willing to accept that responsibility. (+5) O No, I am not yet willing to accept that responsibility. (-5)
3. If you feel that you are in worse shape than when you were younger, to what do you attribute your current physical state of health?	O I think my family history has a lot to do with it. (-1) O It could be because I'm less active now than when I was younger. (+3) O I think it is part of the natural aging process. (-1) O I have no idea why I am in worse shape than when I was younger. (0)

Day 1 - Fitness is a State of Mind

4. During times that you feel tired or run down, would you say it is because you are "getting older," or are you willing and able to accept that it is a result of your lifestyle choices?

○ I would say it is because I am "getting older." (-1)
○ I am willing and able to accept that it is a result of my lifestyle choices. (+3)
○ I attribute it to something else altogether. (-3)

5. Are you currently on any diabetes, high blood pressure, or heart disease medications you were not on when you were younger?

○ Yes, and I want to get off these medications. (+3)
○ Yes, and I am okay with having to take these medications. (-3)
○ No, thankfully I do not have to take any of these medications. (0)

6. In order to achieve your fitness goals, are you willing to dedicate at least 5 hours a week to some form of physical activity?

○ Yes, I am willing to dedicate at least 5 hours a week to some form of physical activity. (+5)
○ No, I am not yet willing to dedicate at least 5 hours a week to some form of physical activity (-5)

7. If waking up a little bit earlier in the morning, and/or staying up a little bit later at night would help you achieve your overall health goals, would you be willing to make those sacrifices?

○ Yes, I would be willing to make those sacrifices. (+5)
○ No, I am not yet willing to make those sacrifices. (-5)

8. Are you willing to join a health club/gym today?

○ Yes, I am willing to join a health club/gym today. (+3)
○ No, I am not yet willing or able to join a health club/gym today. (-3)

9. Are you willing to find a workout partner to help encourage you to exercise regularly?

○ Yes, I am willing to find a workout partner. (+5)
○ No, I do not want, need, or am willing to find a workout partner. (-5)

10. How would you respond if a family member, friend, or someone else you know suggested that because of your past history, you will not be successful in achieving your health goals?	○ I would tell them that my past does not determine my future. (+2) ○ I would tell them I am well aware that I need to make some changes in my life, and I am willing to do whatever it takes. (+5) ○ I would probably start doubting myself. (-5)
11. If there are people in your life who offer little or no support toward helping you achieve for your goals, would you be willing to make some changes in your social circles in order to spend more time with those who do?	○ Yes, I would rather spend time with people who are willing to offer support toward achieving my goals. (+5) ○ No, I am not yet willing to make any changes in my social circles. (-5)
12. Are you willing to have a relaxed, non-confrontational conversation with your family and friends to share your health goals and the steps you plan to take to achieve them?	○ Yes, I am willing to do this as soon as possible. (+5) ○ I am willing, but a little hesitant to do so just yet. (-3) ○ No, I am not willing to share my health goals. (-5)
13. What would you do if an expert presented some information about diet and exercise that is very different from your current beliefs or knowledge?	○ I would keep an open mind about learning something new and/or changing my way of thinking. (+3) ○ I would ask a friend what they thought I should do. (0) ○ I would ignore the advice and just go with what I believe and already know. (-3)
14. If you were told to get rid of all of the unhealthy food in your pantry, refrigerator, and freezer and start over with healthier options would you take this advice?	○ Yes, I am willing to throw away any unhealthy food items in my home. (+5) ○ No, I hate to throw out food. (-5)

Day 1 - Fitness is a State of Mind

Tallying and Interpreting Your Score

Now tally up your score based upon your answers.

16 to 58: Great news!
If you scored between 16 to 58 you are ready and willing to do what it takes to achieve your goals and create an overall healthier lifestyle. Whether you are unhappy with how you look and feel, tired of listening to others who do not support you, or some other reason, you have decided that the buck stops here. Your past will no longer determine your future!

-15 to +15: You are probably experiencing some hesitation or fear.
Making significant changes to the way you have been eating and exercising is not an easy task. It requires a lot of commitment, effort, and trust in the process. However, do not worry. If you are experiencing some hesitation or fear, you are not alone as almost everyone travels down that road at least once along their journey. Those that are successful will tell you the challenges were ultimately worth it and brought them into a great state of overall wellness. You simply need to clarify what you really want in your life then begin taking steps to achieve your goals.

-56 to -16: True transformation begins with taking the first step.
If you scored between -56 to -16 ask yourself these tough questions. Are you really ready to change your life? Are you really sick and tired of gaining weight, taking medications, and/or experiencing negative emotions when you look at yourself in the mirror? Do you really understand that the longer you delay in making significant changes to your eating and exercise habits, the more damage you could be doing to your body? Remember, the purpose of this questionnaire is not to criticize you for your thoughts or actions in the past, rather to discover those areas where you are not quite ready to experience transformation.

Day 2

Goals Propel Purpose

In 2006, I had the honor of hearing Dr. Tony Evans speak at the Kingdom Advisors annual conference. I bought his CD and have listened to this message at least 40 times. Dr. Evans speaks about the difference between a calling and a career. He said,

> "I hope you do what you do as a calling and not simply as career. There is a difference. A career is a job. It is a salary. A calling is a divine reason for doing it. A calling is made up of four fundamental things, **passion, abilities, experiences, and opportunities.** Your calling is always bigger than you. Always! God told Adam and Eve, 'To be fruitful, multiply and fill the whole earth.' That's a pretty big calling. He told Abraham, 'I'm going to make your legacy like the sand of the sea. You are going to father a nation.' That's a pretty big calling. 'Moses, go tell Pharaoh let my people go.' I can't do that. That's a pretty big calling. If your calling you can do, either you do not understand your calling or that ain't it. Because your calling is always bigger than you. It demands God which is why you must serve the purposes of God."

As For Me and My Body

Even with our health and our bodies we must serve the purposes of God. In 1 Corinthians 6:19-20 Paul exclaims, *"Do not you realize that your body is the temple of the Holy Spirit, who lives in you and was given to you by God? You do not belong to yourself, for God bought you with a high price. So you must honor God with your body."*

My prayer is that you are living your dream, fulfilling your calling, or taking the necessary steps to achieve both. I would love to hear from you about how you are progressing on your 21-Day Quest. Send me your questions, share your stories and testimonies.

Day 2
Unlocking My Optimal Performance

Moment of Truth: Even with our health and our bodies we must serve the purposes of God.

Verse to Remember: *"Don't you realize that your body is the temple of the Holy Spirit, who lives in you and was given to you by God? You do not belong to yourself, for God bought you with a high price. So you must honor God with your body."* 1 Corinthians 6:19-20 (NLT)

Challenge to Implement: *Are you fulfilling your life's calling? If so, give thanks for being able to live your purpose. Then, identify two steps you can take to further your calling. If you are not fulfilling your calling, identify two steps you can take towards living God's purpose for your life.*

Soli Deo Gloria and *Arise!*®

Candice

Day 2 - Goals Propel Purpose

Habit, also known as consistency, will either help or hurt your overall health. Many health problems can be traced back to poor habits. Aside from medical conditions that make it challenging to lose weight, poor habits significantly contribute to the obesity crisis that our world faces.

It is time to help you *Arise!*® . The following CMF equation is a key tool we use to empower clients to achieve their wellness goals.

$$\frac{\begin{array}{c}\text{Outcome Goals}\\ \text{- Limiting Factors}\\ \text{+ Behavior Goals}\end{array}}{= \textit{Arise!}^{®}\text{ to a New You}}$$

The first thing you must decide is your outcome goal. Outcome goals are the intended results that will occur from carrying out behaviors. It is a long term measure of strategic effectiveness. One of the key characteristics of an outcome goal is the fact that you cannot directly control the accomplishment of the goal. It is the result of a series of things you must do. For example, an outcome goal could be, losing 12 pounds in 12 weeks, or running a 9-minute mile.

For your goal setting to be optimally effective, you need to define what your goals are and do so systematically. Thus, today you will set SMART goals. Meaning goals that are specific, measurable, attainable, relevant, and time bound. On Day 3, you will analyze what your limiting factors are, and then on Day 4 you will replace those limiting factors with behavior goals. This is how we begin to help you *Arise!*® to a New You!

SMART Goals

Specific	The specificity of goal setting involves answering most of the following questions. • **Why** am I creating this goal? Are there any benefits to carrying out this goal? • **Who** is involved in this goal? Does this goal involve one or more participants? • **What** do I need to accomplish? What outcome or steps to the eventual outcome are desired? • **Where** will I accomplish this goal? Does this goal require a gym? Can I achieve it at home, at work, or throughout my daily activities? Write your goals down. Unwritten or unrecorded goals are nothing more than a wish or dream. Although wishes and dreams are nice, they usually do not come true without a written plan of action. Even better, share your goals with your accountability partner listed in *"My Pledge."*
Measurable	There must be continual objective measurement of your goal behavior to track your progress. • This measurement will help you evaluate whether you are on track in reaching a specific goal and will also show if modifications are necessary to reach the desired goal. You must choose a way to track your progress. Otherwise, the results will be inconclusive. For example, if wearing a size 6 is your goal, an objective measure you can use is your clothes size.

Day 2 - Goals Propel Purpose

Attainable	In goal attainment, it is helpful to evaluate the necessary steps to achieve your goal. Thus, assessing your abilities, skills, and attitudes toward an outcome is critical to determining your goal's attainability. • When a goal is realistic, you are willing to strive toward its accomplishment. • When you believe that you can achieve the goal, the motivation, drive, and perseverance to reach the goal will be available. What is something realistic you want to achieve? Consider making your goals attainable by making them incremental. Taking baby steps creates quick wins which will propel you to keep working towards all your goals.
Relevant	Relevant goals are pertinent to your unique needs, interests, and abilities. • When a goal is relevant, you are motivated to strive toward its achievement. What is going to make you go to the gym on the days you do not want to go? The days when you want to sit on the couch, skipping your workout session? Your goals need to be very inspiring to help you overcome the days you lack motivation. Think creatively and define what will cause you to have unbreakable inner motivation. I always ask clients, why do you want to achieve this now? What is going to make today, this time different? Ask yourself these same questions.

Time-bound	When will the goal be accomplished? • A schedule for the overall goal and the incremental steps behind that goal must be created. It is critical to set a deadline for your goals. Given long-term healthy weight loss is 1-2 pounds per week, it is feasible to want to lose 8 pounds in 10 weeks. I am never going to try to sell you a quick fix gimmick where people lose 20 pounds in 10 days.

Day 2
Unlocking My Optimal Performance

Moment of Truth: Many of the health issues people suffer can be traced back to poor habits.

Quote to Remember: *"Motivation is what gets you started. Habit is what keeps you going."* - Jim Ryun

Challenge to Implement: *Write down one outcome goal for each of the following areas: Overall, Nutrition, Strength training, and Rest..*

Soli Deo Gloria and *Arise!*®

Candice

Day 2 - Goals Propel Purpose

Outcome Goal:

HOW IS MY GOAL SMART?

SPECIFIC

MEASURABLE

TIME-BOUND

ATTAINABLE

RELEVANT

Nutrition Goal:

HOW IS MY GOAL SMART?

SPECIFIC

MEASURABLE

TIME-BOUND

ATTAINABLE

RELEVANT

Day 2 - Goals Propel Purpose

Strength Training Goal:

HOW IS MY GOAL SMART?

SPECIFIC

MEASURABLE

TIME-BOUND

ATTAINABLE

RELEVANT

As For Me and My Body

Rest Goal:

HOW IS MY GOAL SMART?

SPECIFIC

MEASURABLE

TIME-BOUND

ATTAINABLE

RELEVANT

Day 3

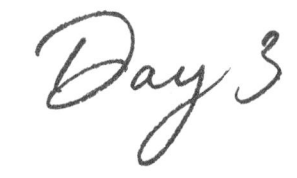

Limiting Factors

In Romans 7:15-16, Paul openly admits his anguish when he says,
> "I don't really understand myself, for I want to do what is right, but I do not do it. Instead, I do what I hate."

In verse 18-19 he continues,
> "I want to do what is right, but I can't. I want to do what is good, but I don't. I don't want to do what is wrong, but I do it anyway."

Paul found himself tormented by his daily struggle with sin. This inward struggle with sin was as real for Paul as it is for us because our flesh and spirit are continuously in constant conflict.

For analogy's sake, many people often experience this same challenge within their own lives when it comes to diet and exercise. Some will say, "I do not really understand myself. I want to lose weight, increase my energy, and improve my physique, but I do not stick to my daily habits and regimen needed to reach my goals. Instead, I eat more and exercise less. I want to eat right and exercise, but I cannot. I want to live a healthy lifestyle, but I do not.

I do not want my physique to continue to be this size and shape, but I never take action or follow through with a long-term plan."

Fortunately for Paul and all believers in Christ, he found peace. All believers who realize the truth in Romans 8:2,
> "And because you belong to Him, the power of the life giving Spirit has freed you from the power of sin that leads to death."

have the power of the Holy Spirit to conquer all inward struggles, including living a healthy lifestyle and most importantly, sin.

Day 3
Unlocking My Optimal Performance

Moment of Truth: Believers have the Holy Spirit to conquer all inward struggles, including living a healthy lifestyle and most importantly, sin.

Verse to Remember: *"And because you belong to Him, the power of the life giving Spirit has freed you from the power of sin that leads to death."*

Romans 8:2 (NLT)

Challenge to Implement: *Think about and identify the limiting factors that are keeping you from complete unison with God.*

Soli Deo Gloria and *Arise!*®

Candice

Day 3 - Limiting Factors

Do you want to achieve great results? Then you must master your limiting factors. Anything that prevents you from achieving optimal results is a limiting factor. Identifying your limiting factors enables you to overcome them. When you master your limiting factors, you exude a can-do attitude that boosts your confidence and motivates you to commit to your fitness. We all have weaknesses. When we understand those weaknesses, we can immediately identify what holds us back, what limits our success.

Take a moment to consider your current habits. How is your eating? Are you getting sufficient hours of sleep? How active are you? Which of these areas need improvement? What is limiting you from improving them? Is your environment conducive to your success? What types of messages flood your mind regularly as you browse social media or watch television? Change begins within. Are you mentally prepared to do what is necessary to commit to a new, better version of you? Do you have a healthy support circle to encourage and help hold you accountable? All of this is important.

While change begins with you, research has shown people with a strong support network thrive. Having a strong social network not only helps with accountability, it also helps to encourage during the most difficult parts of your journey. Our circles have a lot to do with who we are and who we become.

Common Limiting Factors

Mentally unprepared for change	Poor food choices at home and when dining out
Pantry full of temptation	Little to no food prep due to busy schedule/lack of time

No support or fitness buddy	Frequent travel
Skipping breakfast	Social activities consume large portion of time
Uncommitted	Bored with food

Set yourself up for success, do not attempt to address all your limiting factors at once. Instead, select a complementary few to work on simultaneously. For example, if poor food selections are a big limiting factor, tackle it first. Complement it with clearing out your kitchen. Eliminate unhealthy foods and replace them with healthy alternatives. Then, commit to preparing your meals instead of eating out frequently. As your commitment becomes habit, begin to add other limiting factors.

Day 3
Unlocking My Optimal Performance

Moment of Truth: To achieve great results, you only need to master one crucial skill: The ability to know your limiting factors and remove them!

Quote to Remember: "Build up your weaknesses until they become your strong points." - Knute Rockne

Challenge to Implement: Review your score and interpretation from the Readiness for Change questionnaire you completed Day 1. Then complete and score the Social Support and Kitchen Questionnaire below. Finally, after completing and interpreting the questionnaires, write down your biggest limiting factor in the areas of: mental readiness for change, social support and your kitchen environment.

Soli Deo Gloria and *Arise!*®

Candice

Day 3 - Limiting Factors

Limiting Factors

My biggest mental readiness limiting factor is:

My biggest social support limiting is:

My biggest environmental limiting factor is:

Social Support Questionnaire

The Social Support Questionnaire is designed to help you make an honest assessment of your level of social support – the people surrounding you on a daily or regular basis.

Whether trusted family members, friends, co-workers, acquaintances from clubs, church, or other organizations – or a combination thereof–a strong social support network can provide mental, emotional, and/or tangible assistance and encouragement in both the good and challenging times. Community, security, and a sense of belonging are the major benefits of a strong social support network and have been proven to help enhance one's quality of life.

On the flip side, the absence of a strong social support network can be detrimental to your physical, mental, and emotional health and can make it difficult to accomplish your goals.

One note: Be honest. The purpose of this questionnaire is not to judge others for their actions or inactions in support of your healthy lifestyle goals. Rather it is to discover any areas where a few tweaks to your social support network may be more beneficial. So let us take a close, but loving look at the current people and situations surrounding you.

Question	Response and Scoring
1. Does your spouse or significant other engage in healthy lifestyle habits including eating healthy, exercising regularly, and getting adequate sleep?	O Yes, my spouse/significant other engages in healthy lifestyle habits. (+5) O No, my spouse/significant other does not engage in healthy lifestyle habits. (-5) O I currently do not have a spouse or significant other. (0)

Day 3 - Limiting Factors

2. Other than your spouse or significant other, do the people you are around most of the time such as at work and home engage in healthy lifestyle habits including eating healthy, exercising regularly, and getting adequate sleep?

   ○ Yes, most of them engage in healthy lifestyle habits. (+3)
   ○ About half of them engage in healthy lifestyle habits. (0)
   ○ No, most of them do not engage in healthy lifestyle habits. (-3)

3. Does anyone you live with bring nourishing, wholesome foods beneficial to our bodies into your home?

   ○ When bringing home food, they always choose healthy options. (+5)
   ○ They sometimes bring home healthy options. (0)
   ○ No, they never bring home healthy options. (-5)

4. On the other side of the coin, does anyone you live with bring any foods that are not beneficial to our bodies into your home?

   ○ Yes, they always bring home foods that are not beneficial to our bodies. (-5)
   ○ They sometimes bring home foods that are not beneficial to our bodies. (-3)
   ○ No, they never bring home foods that are not beneficial to our bodies. (0)

5. When at work do your coworkers tend to bring in lots of unhealthy snacks like candy, cookies, donuts, chips, etc.?

   ○ Yes, my coworkers tend to bring in lots of unhealthy snacks. (-4)
   ○ Yes, but not very often. (0)
   ○ No, my coworkers never bring in unhealthy snacks. (+4)

As For Me and My Body

6. When dining out, do your companions choose healthy, nourishing options?
   - ○ Yes, they always choose healthy, nourishing options. (+2)
   - ○ Yes, but only about half of the time. (0)
   - ○ No, they never choose nourishing, wholesome options. (-2)

7. When discussing your overall healthy lifestyle goals with friends, family, or others do they seem interested in learning more or possibly joining you? Or do they tend to brush you off and dismiss your goals?
   - ○ They generally seem interested in learning more or possibly joining me. (+2)
   - ○ They do not seem interested in learning more or joining me. (0)
   - ○ They brush me off or dismiss my goals. (-2)

8. Do you feel that those around you support achieving your healthy goals by sharing exercise, dietary, or other healthy lifestyle information with you?
   - ○ Yes, they always support me by sharing healthy lifestyle information. (+5)
   - ○ They sometimes support me by sharing healthy lifestyle information. (+2)
   - ○ No, they never support me by sharing healthy lifestyle information. (0)

9. Do you belong to a health club/gym where you typically work out at least 3 times a week?
   - ○ Yes, and on average I have been working out there at least 3 times a week for at least 1 year. (+2)
   - ○ I belong to a health club/gym, but I just recently joined. (+1)
   - ○ No, I do not belong to a health club/gym. (0)

Day 3 - Limiting Factors

10. Other than at a health club/gym, are you a member of any recreational teams, clubs, or groups that meet at least 2 times a week?
    - ○ Yes, and I have been a member for at least 1 year (+5)
    - ○ I am a member of a recreational team, club, or group, but I just recently joined. (+2)
    - ○ No, I do not belong to a recreational team, club, or group. (0)

11. Do the people you live or work with tend to plan activities that conflict with your regular exercise schedule?
    - ○ Yes, they seem to always plan schedule activities that conflict with my regular exercise schedule. (-3)
    - ○ Sometimes, but I do not think it's intentional. (-1)
    - ○ No. They understand how important my exercise routine is to me. (+3)

12. Is it easy to find someone to join you for a walk, hike, bike ride, or some other kind of physical activity?
    - ○ Yes, it is easy to find someone to join me for some kind of physical activity. (+2)
    - ○ No, most people I know are not interested in physical activity. (-2)

Tallying and Interpreting Your Score

Now tally up your score based upon the answers you gave above.

20 to 38 total points: Congratulations!

If you scored between 20 to 38 points, you are blessed to have a great social support network around you, and it plays an integral role in helping you achieve your healthy lifestyle goals. Another added benefit is that because you feel supported, you naturally desire to support others in achieving their goals as well, so you are definitely living on "a two-way street!"

5 to 19 points: It is good but could be better.
There appears to be a somewhat good social support network around you, but there are also areas where you are experiencing challenges. The good thing is that you now have some insight into where you may want or need to make changes that align with your vision and goals.

-14 to 4 points: Needs Improvement.
A score between -14 to 4 points indicates there are some areas in your social circles that support your goals, but most of them do not. However, this is not always attributed to the people currently around you, rather the opportunities to encounter those people, which only you can create. By joining a team, club, or other recreational group, or even signing up for a gym membership, you will meet others who have a similar interest in physical fitness. Consequently, establishing a friendship with them will naturally strengthen your social support network.

-31 to -15 points: You have a lot of work to do.
The purpose of this questionnaire is not to judge others for their actions or inactions in support of your healthy lifestyle goals but to help you establish a strong social support network. Remember, this takes time and effort. One helpful step is to have a relaxed, non-confrontational conversation with your family, friends and co-workers to help them understand how important their love and support is to you. Share with them your dreams, goals and desires, and the steps you plan to take to achieve them. Ask if they would be willing to join you on a walk, for a nutritious meal, or to check out a potential new gym or recreational activity. You may be surprised to learn you have some common interests neither of you knew about! This may be a little difficult at first, but do not give up. You are worth it!

Day 3 - Limiting Factors

Kitchen Makeover Questionnaire

The Kitchen Makeover Questionnaire is designed to help you make an honest assessment of your current situation, as well as guide you forward in making better, healthier food and lifestyle choices.

The foundation of any healthy eating program is, of course, the food you put into your body. In addition to getting plenty of exercise, rest, fresh air, and sunshine the healthier the food you put in, the better you will look and feel.

But before you start shopping for all that great healthy food, it is very important to take stock of what you already have on hand to determine what stays and what goes. Sorry, but those deliciously decadent French macarons dipped in dark chocolate are not going to make the cut!

One note: Be honest. This is not meant to be a judgement on what you have done in the past, rather a place of reflection on where you are now so you can set an intention for the good health and happiness you would like to experience in the future.

Question	Response and Scoring

1. Do you have the following items in your pantry?

Healthy Pantry List
- Canned or bagged beans
- Extra virgin olive oil
- Natural peanut butter (made with peanuts only, or only peanuts and salt)
- Mixed nuts
- Quinoa
- Whole grain pastas (buckwheat, couscous, brown rice, etc.)
- Whole oats
- Vinegar (white, red, apple cider, rice wine, etc.)
- Green tea
- Supplements (protein, green foods, fish oil, etc.)

○ I have all of these items in my pantry. (+5)
○ I have more than half of these items in my pantry. (+2)
○ I have less than half of these items in my pantry. (-2)
○ I do not have any of these items in my pantry. (-5)

Unhealthy Pantry List
- Conventional peanut butter (contains sugar and hydrogenated vegetable oil for smooth consistency)
- Cookies (regular or low-fat)
- Chips (corn or potato)
- Crackers (club, saltine, graham, etc.)
- Dried bread products (breadcrumbs, croutons, etc.)
- Instant Foods (noodles, rice, mashed potatoes, hot cereals, powdered items, etc.)
- Fruit or granola bars
- Candy or chocolates
- Soft drinks (diet or regular sodas, flavored waters, and other sweetened drinks)
- Four or more types of alcohol (wine, beer, spirits, hard liquors, etc.)

○ I have all of these items in my pantry. (-5)
○ I have more than half of these items in my pantry. (-2)
○ I have less than half of these items in my pantry. (+2)
○ I do not have any of these items in my pantry. (+5)

Day 3 - Limiting Factors

2. Do you have the following items in your refrigerator or freezer?

Healthy Refrigerator or Freezer List
- Fruit (at least three different varieties)
- Vegetables (at least three different varieties)
- Sweet potatoes
- Beef (extra-lean)
- Salmon
- Chicken (breasts)
- Flaxseed oil
- Natural cheeses (non-pasteurized)
- Eggs or packaged egg whites

○ I have all of these items in my refrigerator or freezer. (+5)
○ I have more than half of these items in my refrigerator or freezer. (+2)
○ I have less than half of these items in my refrigerator or freezer. (-2)
○ I do not have any of these items in my refrigerator or freezer. (-5)

Unhealthy Pantry List
- Baked goods
- Margarine or butter
- Fruit juice
- High fat meats (beef, sausage, hot dogs, corned beef, salami, etc.)
- Sauces (gravy, hollandaise, mayonnaise or cream based, etc.)
- Leftovers (from a restaurant meal or take-out place)
- Frozen dinners (all kinds)

○ I have all of these items in my refrigerator or freezer. (-5)
○ I have more than half of these items in my refrigerator or freezer. (-2)
○ I have less than half of these items in my refrigerator or freezer. (+2)
○ I do not have any of these items in my refrigerator or freezer. (+5)

3. **Do you have snack foods like chips, crackers, candy, etc. in plain view?**
   - ○ Yes, they are out where I can see them. (-5)
   - ○ No, they are hidden from view. (+5)

4. **In general, how often do you go grocery shopping?**
   - ○ About once a week (+1)
   - ○ More than once a week (+5)
   - ○ Less than 3 times a month (-5)

5. **Do you buy foods in larger, economy-sized bags/containers, or in standard smaller sizes?**
   - ○ More than half of the time I buy foods in larger, economy-sized bags/containers. (-3)
   - ○ More than half of the time I buy foods in standard smaller sizes. (+3)

6. **Do you prepare meals in advance (for school, work, when out and about, travel, etc.?)**
   - ○ I always prepare meals in advance. (+5)
   - ○ More than half of the time I prepare meals in advance. (+2)
   - ○ Less than half of the time I prepare meals in advance. (-2)
   - ○ I never prepare meals in advance. (-5)

Day 3 – Limiting Factors

7. When you follow recipes when preparing meals, do you tend to choose healthy recipes?

   ○ Yes, I choose healthy recipes most of the time. (+5)
   ○ I choose healthy recipes about half of the time. (0)
   ○ No, I never choose healthy recipes. (-5)

8. Can you identify whether each of the foods in your home are composed of mostly proteins, carbohydrates, or fats?

   ○ Yes, I am aware of the different components of the food in my home. (+2)
   ○ No, I do not know what makes up the food in my home. (-2)

9. Do you think "healthy eating" means adhering to a low-fat diet?

   ○ Yes (-2)
   ○ No (+2)

10. When you have guests in your home, do you buy or prepare healthy food options, or what you think they will like or want?

    ○ I buy or prepare healthy food options. (+3)
    ○ I buy or prepare what I think they will like or want. (-3)

11. Whether or not you purchased it, someone brought it to your home, or it was sent as a gift, are you hesitant to throw out food that no longer fits your healthy eating plan?

    ○ Yes, I hate to throw out food. (-5)
    ○ Sometimes, but more than half of the time I will throw it out. (0)
    ○ No, I am willing to throw away any unhealthy food items in my home. (+5)

12. Do you have the following items in your kitchen?

- Food processor
- Blender
- Non-toxic/environmentally friendly pots and pans
- Non-toxic/environmentally friendly food containers
- Non-toxic/environmentally friendly utensils (spatulas, cooking spoons, knives, fruit and vegetable peelers, etc.)
- Portable bottles for shakes, smoothies and other healthy beverages
- Water filter (built into the refrigerator, or a movable one like a Brita, etc.)
- Tea kettle
- Food scale
- Portable cooler for meals on-the-go

○ I have all of these items in my kitchen. (+5)
○ I have more than half of these items in my kitchen. (+2)
○ I have less than half of these items in my kitchen. (-2)
○ I do not have any of these items in my kitchen. (-5)

Tallying and Interpreting Your Score

Now tally up your score based upon the answers you gave above.

29 to 60 points: Excellent work!
If you scored between 29 to 60 points, you do not need much of a makeover. A quick review of your answers will let you know which adjustments are needed to raise your score.

2 to 28 points: Nice job
You are doing a nice job and only need to make a few minor tweaks. Perhaps you need to add a few kitchen utensils or throw out those last packages of cookies and chips. Maybe branching out with a little more variety in the fruit and/or

Day 3 - Limiting Factors

vegetable department will do the trick. Whatever it is, you can do it! Just a few more steps…

-28 to 1 points: Needs Improvement
Well, things are not bleak, but there is definitely room for improvement. People who score between -28 to 1 point often find that the needed adjustments are to increase their kitchen appliances and related items (See #12), and to **add** more foods from the Healthy pantry and Healthy refrigerator and freezer lists (See #1 and #2, respectively). You will most likely also need to **decrease or eliminate altogether** those listed in the Unhealthy pantry and Unhealthy refrigerator and freezer lists (Also in #1 and #2, respectively).

-60 to -29 points: You have some work to do
If you scored between -60 to -29 points, do not despair. Again, this is not meant to be a judgement on what you have done in the past, rather a place of reflection on where you are now so you can set an intention for the good health and happiness you would like to experience in the future. Not sure where to start? A few suggestions might be to begin using healthy recipes instead of making it up as you go, learning more about the structure of the foods we eat to help make better choices, or preparing meals in advance when on the go, just to name a few. Once you get going, you will look so good your family and friends will want to know what you are doing!

Day 4

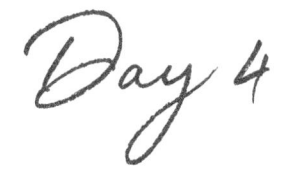

Behavioral Goals

I love autobiographies, and one of my favorite autobiographies is, *"Extraordinary, Ordinary People,"* by Condoleezza Rice. From this incredible read, I took away four things:

1. **Never wonder or have regrets.** Secretary Rice contemplated whether she should get her PhD. For me, Thunderbird School of Global Management was always my dream school. Reading her book made me think about this dream I had shelved, inspiring me to fulfill my dream of attending Thunderbird.

2. **Be at the top of your industry.** Embrace your natural abilities and passions so that you naturally become the "best" in your industry. Secretary Rice loves to play the piano, but she realized that she would never be exceptional like some others. I am a numbers person. Math was always an easier subject for me, but naturally I have been an athlete since I was 3 years old. The decision to leave finance, step into the world of health and wellness, and never look back was one of the best decisions I have made. As I walked out of Merrill Lynch for the last time, I distinctly remember the quiet voice speaking to me saying, "Candice do not look back." Eleven years later I am continuing to only look forward in

the health and wellness industry.

3. **Make tough decisions.** When Secretary Rice was asked what she thought Stanford's greatest challenge was, she replied,
   > "I answered that the university had strayed from its core purposes and was trying to do too much. Across-the-board budget cuts threatened academic programs and social activities almost equally. I used an example from my time in the Pentagon grappling with priority setting. 'Whenever you ask the Joint Chiefs of Staff a question about what to cut, the answer is one-third of a tank, one-third of an aircraft, and one-third of a ship. That's how the university seems to work too. Everything is equal. No one is prepared to make hard choices."

   The first company I co-created was also in the health and wellness industry. I dedicated five great years and loved how much I learned about business and entrepreneurship. Deciding to walk away was one of the toughest decisions I have ever made, but I knew my calling was taking me in a new direction.

4. **Make sacrifices.** Like everything else in our lives, we must dedicate time and formulate a game plan. Secretary Rice once said something that grabbed my attention, "Books do not write themselves." It took me five years to get serious about writing this book, accomplishing this major goal on my "Things to do in Life List." I am glad I did and I hope you are too!

God uses ordinary people to achieve extraordinary things. Think about it. Moses was a total failure as the prince of Egypt, and God called him to deliver a nation. When Goliath was taunting the Israelites, everyone discounted David, a teenage shepherd boy, but God did not! David then defeated the giant and became the king of a nation. Nehemiah, was serving as a cup-bearer and God called him to rebuild the walls around Jerusalem. Mary was a teenage girl when God called her to be the mother of the Messiah. Simon Peter would have lived

Day 4 - Behavioral Goals

and died an ordinary fisherman except Jesus called him to establish the church. Isaiah was a scribe in the royal place in Jerusalem, which was a respectable career. But God had other plans for his servant. Isaiah became, and is considered, the greatest prophet.

God uses improbable men and women, like you and me, who have nothing of our own to offer, except our faithfulness and willingness to say, "Yes." While writing this book, I wrestled with the thought of failure and ineptness. In my mind, I would say, "Lord I can't do this as I fall daily. I'm not good enough…I do not know the bible enough…I'm clueless about how I will draw parallel connections between one's physical health and spiritual walk." In other words, I made excuse after excuse. The struggle was real but the power of prayer is even more real. I dedicated quiet time, faithfully read, and studied the Word of God - I had to be still to write. He is calling us right now. When He calls, will you be like Isaiah and say, "Send me"?

Day 4
Unlocking My Optimal Performance

Moment of Truth: God uses flawed people to achieve extraordinary things. Just like you, just like me.

Verse to Remember: *"Then I heard the Lord asking, 'Whom should I send as messenger to this people? Who will go for us?' I said, 'Here I am. Send me.'"*

Isaiah 6:8 (NLT)

Challenge to Implement: *Meditate on how God uses ordinary people to do the extraordinary. Even more importantly, how you are one of them! Out of the four points, never have regrets, be the top of your industry, make tough decisions, and make sacrifices, pick one to start applying to your life today.*

Soli Deo Gloria and *Arise!*®

Candice

Congratulations! You have identified your Limiting Factors. Now that you know what prevents you from achieving your goals, it is time to define what you can do to overcome those limits. The way to move beyond your Limiting Factors is to replace current behaviors with newer, more positive ones. For each limiting factor you listed, identify a new action you can take to replace it. These new action steps are your Behavior Goals; the steps required to accomplish your goals.

Consider your Behavior Goals carefully. These must be action steps you can commit to performing regularly, as they are directly tied to your goal outcome. If exercise is something new to you, one Behavior Goal may be to learn the proper way to execute all of the moves you plan to incorporate before beginning. This reduces your risk of injury and also increases the likelihood of your sticking to the activity. If your goal is to eat healthier, then perhaps your behavior goal is to add an additional 2-3 servings more of fresh fruit and vegetables. No matter your desired outcome, you must establish a set of behaviors.

Day 3
Unlocking My Optimal Performance

Moment of Truth: Behavioral Goals are the actions you can directly control.

Quote to Remember: *"Behavior is what a man does, not what he thinks, feels, or believes." - Anonymous*

Challenge to Implement: *The behavior goals you establish must be based on your limiting factors. Review your biggest limiting factor in the areas of mental readiness for change, social support, and your kitchen environment (identified in Day 3). Then write down a corresponding behavior goal that can help you overcome the limiting factors you identified. Additionally, write down other behavior goals you must implement to achieve the overall outcome goal(s) you set in Day 2.*

Soli Deo Gloria and *Arise!*®

Candice

Day 4 - Behavioral Goals

Behavior Goals

To overcome my mental readiness limiting factor, the behavior goal I will implement is:

To overcome my social support limiting factor, the behavior goal I will implement is:

To overcome my environmental limiting factor, the behavior goal I will implement is:

To achieve my overall outcome goal, other behavior goals I will implement are:

Day 5

Balancing Energy

My paternal grandmother lived to be 96 years young! Sharp as a whistle and with unbelievable wit, her charisma, her love for life, people, family, and most importantly, Christ, shined daily. This is despite living the last 10 years or so of her life with no sight in one eye and very little in the other. One of her favorite things she would do was take her trusted magnifying glass and read the Bible. At some point I started reading the Bible to her on my visits. It was special. We would lie in her twin bed, I would read, and she would listen or sometimes snore. This ritual expanded to me calling her every night to read the Bible to her. Our daily readings went on for about 2 years and it truly was a privilege and honor to read to her the book that gives energy, life, and sustains us. One night after I was reading, she broke out in the sweetest, "thank you, thank you, thank you," that I ever heard. I captured it in my journal entry and it reads:

> Thursday, May 5, 2011 @ 11:20pm.
> *"I pray I always remember Granny's voice as she said the 3 thank yous! It was so genuine, sincere and loving as if she was a kid resting on Jesus' chest thanking Him like she was not going to ever have a chance to thank Him again."*

Although, she no longer had eyesight to read, the source of her energy and strength was still the Word of God. The memories and joy I received from reading to her are priceless.

In the book, *Walking by Faith* by Jennifer Rothschild, she speaks about a time someone asked her, "If you could see for a day or a moment, what would you want to see?" Her response has always stayed with me as it reminded me of my grandmother. She stated she would simply want the opportunity to see the words in the Bible and read them. WOW! We often forget the simplest things in life, like the privilege of having and being able to use our five senses! I know my grandmother would have wished for this same gift. Before complaining about having to exercise or eat healthier, pause for a second and cherish the fact that you can work out, and that you can eat healthier. Unfortunately, there are millions of people across the world who dream that they could simply go workout, feed themselves and perform the daily tasks we often take for granted.

Day 5
Unlocking My Optimal Performance

Moment of Truth: The source of our energy and strength is the Word of God.

Verse to Remember: *"But those who trust in the Lord will find new strength. They will soar high on wings like eagles. They will run and not grow weary. They will walk and not faint."*
Isaiah 40:31 (NLT)

Challenge to Implement: *Begin reading the Word daily, as it truly is the source of our energy. If you are doing this already then which of the five senses are you taking for granted? Furthermore, using this sense how can you bless someone who lacks this sense?*

Soli Deo Gloria and *Arise!*

Candice

Day 5 - Balancing Energy

Have you ever wondered how and why various weight loss plans can all produce successful results? The answer lies in understanding energy balance as it is the most important determining factor of your weight loss, gain, or maintenance progress. The common denominator between all successful weight loss plans, whether it is low carb, high protein, high fat, etc., is that a negative energy balance is established. Hence, following any nutrition plan typically leads to calorie control.

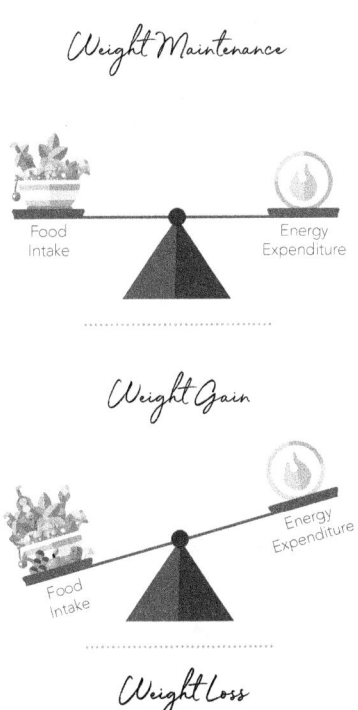

Weight Maintenance

Weight Gain

Weight Loss

Unfortunately, as adults we often like to make things complex and complicated, especially when it comes to our nutrition. The reality is if your goal is weight loss, you must expend more energy than you consume, or establish a negative energy balance. Burn more calories than you eat; when your energy expenditure outweighs your food intake, you lose weight. If your goal is to gain weight, you simply need to create a positive energy balance. When your food intake outweighs your expenditure, you gain weight.

Energy balance is the relationship between energy intake, more commonly referred to as food intake, and energy expenditure. Picture a seesaw with food intake on one end and energy expenditure on the other. If food intake is equal to energy expenditure, weight is maintained. If food intake is greater than energy expenditure, weight is gained. If food intake is less than energy expenditure, weight is lost.

The ideal way to establish a negative energy balance is to increase exercise to at least five hours per week, eat clean 90% of the time, and eat smaller meals throughout the day. Some examples of eating clean throughout the day follow.

Day 5 - Balancing Energy

		Workout in the Morning	Workout in the Morning
Meal One	Protein	2 egg whites; turkey bacon	natural peanut butter - 1tsp
	Veggie/Fruit	onion	
	Starchy Carb	whole wheat grain toast	1 slice wheat bread
	Fat	egg yolk, turkey bacon	natural peanut butter
Meal Two	Protein	turkey from deli	2 egg whites, 1 whole egg
	Veggie/Fruit	strawberries	spinach, kale
	Starchy Carb	oatmeal	oatmeal
	Fat	turkey	yolk from egg
Meal Three	Protein	salmon	smoked salmon (size of hand)
	Veggie/Fruit	zucchini	salad/grapes
	Starchy Carb		
	Fat	olive oil	salad dressing - vinaigrette
Meal Four	Protein	turkey	almonds (15), string cheese
	Veggie/Fruit	apple; celery	red & yellow peppers
	Starchy Carb		
	Fat	natural peanut butter	almonds, 2 string cheese
Meal Five	Protein	ground turkey	rotisserie chicken, steak (size of palm)
	Veggie/Fruit	lettuce, green beans	broccoli
	Starchy Carb		
	Fat	avocado	olive oil

		Workout in the Evening	Workout in the Evening
Meal One	Protein	2 egg whites, 1 whole egg	2 egg whites + 1 whole egg
	Veggie/Fruit	bell peppers	leafy greens (spinach, kale or spring greens)
	Starchy Carb	oatmeal	1 slice wheat bread
	Fat	egg yolk	egg yolk
Meal Two	Protein	greek yogurt	protein powder
	Veggie/Fruit	fresh berries	leafy greens and fruit
	Starchy Carb		
	Fat	greek yogurt	1 tsp natural peanut butter
Meal Three	Protein	chicken breast	peppered turkey breast
	Veggie/Fruit	spinach and romaine lettuce	grapes
	Starchy Carb		
	Fat	chicken breast	2 sticks of string cheese
Meal Four	Protein	natural peanut butter	1 tsp natural peanut butter
	Veggie/Fruit	celery	celery
	Starchy Carb		5 saltine wheat crackers or unsalted tops or 2 rice cakes (unsalted, plain)
	Fat	natural peanut butter	natural peanut butter
Meal Five	Protein	chicken breast	chicken breast
	Veggie/Fruit	broccoli	broccoli
	Starchy Carb	brown rice	sweet potatoes w/ cinnamon and nutmeg only
	Fat	chicken breast	extra virgin olive oil; chicken breast

Day 5 - Balancing Energy

Day 5
Unlocking My Optimal Performance

Moment of Truth: The common denominator between all successful weight loss plans, whether it is a low carb, high protein, high fat, etc., is that a negative energy balance is established!

Quote to Remember: *"Don't diet. Eat according to your goals."* - Anonymous

Challenge to Implement: *Identify your energy balance goal. Then list three daily behavioral goals you will do to achieve your desired energy balance.*

Soli Deo Gloria and *Arise!*®

Candice

Energy Balance

My goal is to establish a _____ energy balance.
(negative, positive or neutral)

To obtain this energy balance, three daily behavioral goals I commit to are:

Example: I will do aerobic exercise for at least 30 minutes a day, or I will follow my nutritional plan with 90% accuracy).

1)

2) _____

3) _____

Day 6

Sky-high Metabolism

On April 8, 2008 when I worked at Merrill Lynch, I received an email from a business acquaintance with the subject titled "Business testimony.":

"Hi Candice:

Knowing that you are a person of faith, I wanted to take the opportunity to respond to your statement that you hoped my business was going well. I struggled many years in a solo practice. I slowly built it up to where I was doing pretty well, all by the Lord's hand and him opening doors.

I told you I have been a Pastor of a church for the past 1.5 years and I have 6 mos. to go. I spend an inordinate amount of time doing church work at my office and wondered if I would be able to keep up financially because I spend entire days just handling church matters. My testimony is that in 2006 I stayed about the same financially; but in 2007 I made more than in any year previous. No way that happens but by the Lord's goodness. Even greater, I had referred a high dollar case to another group of attorneys over 2 years ago because I lacked the expertise and funds to litigate it. Amazingly, it recently settled and I received a portion of the settlement last month that was about as much as I normally net in a year. God is good when you try to do His work and put the Kingdom first (although I fail at that daily) but I'm trying to be faithful and He certainly has been to me. I have not lacked for anything and I have made more in my practice since I took on the "full time" job of Pastor too. I would be remiss if I didn't share that with you. God bless and keep Him first!"

Metabolism breaks down the energy we get from food and turns it into fuel for our bodies to function. Just as our energy must be broken down to provide us with the fuel needed to build us back up, life's challenges do the same. In Romans 5:3-5, Paul offers a great example of this when he states:

"We can rejoice, too, when we run into problems and trials, for we know that they help us develop endurance. And endurance develops strength of character, and character strengthens our confident hope of salvation. And this hope does not lead to disappointment."

Encouraging someone can motivate them with the energy, confidence, and courage they need to simply take one more step or try one more time. Positive energy is infectious, and it truly is a joy to brighten someone's day.

Day 6 - Sky-high Metabolism

> ## Day 6
> ### Unlocking My Optimal Performance
>
> **Moment of Truth:** God is good when you try to do His work and put the Kingdom first.
>
> **Verse to Remember:** *"We can rejoice, too, when we run into problems and trials, for we know that they help us develop endurance. And endurance develops strength of character, and character strengthens our confident hope of salvation. And this hope does not lead to disappointment."*
> *Romans 5:3-5 (NLT)*
>
> **Challenge to Implement:** Send an email, a card or quick note to someone you feel led to share an encouraging word with.
>
> Soli Deo Gloria and *Arise!*®
>
> *Candice*

Ignorance is not bliss. Repeatedly people tell me, my diet is great as I only eat once a day. Immediately, my heart sinks, especially for those who have been doing this for years. More than likely, they have completely destroyed their metabolism. Understand that eating once a day is doing your body more harm than good because our bodies are designed to survive. When you do not eat small meals throughout the day your body does not know when it will receive its next meal. Therefore, when you do finally eat, instead of burning those calories, your body will store them as fat instead. **You cannot outsmart your body's desire to survive.** Your body cannot tell the difference between true starvation and self imposed dietary restriction and both methods will cause it to shut down.

Metabolism is what breaks down the energy you get from food and turns it into fuel for your body to function. Gaining weight means you consume more energy than your metabolism can process. Consequently, you store the unused fuel as fat. This is your body's natural response to excess. Remember, your body cannot distinguish between starvation and self-imposed dietary restriction. Hence, in times of famine, your body holds on to your fat as a protective reserve of energy in order to guarantee your survival. Do not allow yourself to be bamboozled. Eating one meal a day is detrimental to your body's metabolism.

If you have dieted for years, gaining and losing the same weight over and over again, chances are high that you have impacted your metabolism negatively. As a result, your body now burns fuel from food energy at a slow rate, making it very difficult to lose weight.

Day 6 - Sky-high Metabolism

Ways You Can Sabotage Your Body

Yo-Yo Dieting
- Extreme fluctuations in weight loss/weight gain because of yo-yo dieting is unhealthy and unsafe.
- Your metabolism is programmed to operate in feast or famine mode according to what food sources are available.
- Skipping meals triggers a food scarcity response in your body by slowing your metabolism. This response triggers your body to store excess fat.
- Commit to consistent clean eating; make it a lifestyle.

Eliminating Food Groups
- Drastically reducing or eliminating specific food groups (e.g., carbohydrates) can trigger adverse reactions.
- Any weight loss achieved may not last once you reintroduce the food group.
- Eliminating food groups deprives your body of vital nutrients.
- Oftentimes, reintroducing eliminated foods back into your diet results in your body rapidly gaining weight.
- Aim to create a healthy balance of protein, complex carbohydrates, and healthy fats.

Fortunately, metabolism can be retrained to function efficiently even after long periods of dieting.

How to Speed Up Your Metabolism

Resistance Train Regularly	- Muscle burns more calories than fat
- Resistance training releases testosterone into your body which works to destroy fat
Focus on HIIT (high intensity interval training)	- HIIT is repeated spurts of short duration, high-intensity intervals combined with periods of lower intensity intervals of active recovery. Examples of HIIT:
- Jog 30 seconds, then walk 1 minute
- Sprint 30 seconds, then walk 1.5 minutes
- Perform a strength training exercise for 45 seconds, then rest for 1 minute
Eat Clean	Clean eating is a lifestyle:
1. Eat 5-7 smalls meals each day; every 2-3 hours.
2. Eat breakfast every day.
3. Eat a combination of lean protein, healthy fat, and vegetables or fruit with each meal.
4. Eat 2-3 servings of complex carbohydrates (ex. whole grains, sweet potatoes) daily.
5. Consume a minimum of 3 liters of water daily.
6. Pack your prepared meals daily.
7. Consume correct portion sizes.

Committing to clean eating at least 90% of the time will produce significant physical transformations without you denying yourself. |

Day 6 - Sky-high Metabolism

Consume Protein	Because protein is harder to digest, it speeds up your metabolism.
Eliminate these Roadblocks	1. Bypass all processed and refined simple carbs (e.g., potato chips, cookies, crackers, candy) 2. Avoid processed grains, processed flours, and foods with added sugar. 3. Avoid preservatives. 4. Avoid artificial sugars. 5. Avoid saturated and trans fats. 6. Avoid artificial foods (ex. processed cheese slices). 7. Avoid chemically charged foods. 8. Avoid sugary beverages, including soda and fruit juices. 9. Avoid and/or limit alcohol intake. 10. Avoid foods containing little or no nutritional value.

As For Me and My Body

Day 6
Unlocking My Optimal Performance

Moment of Truth: The body cannot tell the difference between true starvation and self imposed dietary restriction. It shuts down either way.

Quote to Remember: "People tend to think that metabolism is genetically predetermined. That you are either cursed or you are blessed. And that's not true." - Jillian Michaels

Challenge to Implement: Out of the five ways identified to speed up your metabolism, pick two to focus on.

Soli Deo Gloria and *Arise!*

Candice

The two ways I will speed up my metabolism are:

1)

2)

Day 7

Sleep to Live

Years ago, I visited the church of a friend of mine, who happened to also be the pastor. That Sunday, he preached from Mark 4:35-41 and brought a powerful message I have always remembered.

> "As evening came Jesus said to his disciples, **'Let's cross to the other side of the lake.'** So they took Jesus in the boat and started out, leaving the crowds behind (although other boats followed). But soon a fierce storm came up. High waves were breaking into the boat and it began to fill with water.
>
> Jesus was sleeping at the back of the boat with his head on a cushion. The disciples woke him up, shouting, 'Teacher do not you care that we're going to drown?' When Jesus woke up he rebuked the wind and said to the water, 'Silence! Be still!' Suddenly the wind stopped, and there was a great calm. Then he asked them, 'Why are you afraid? Do you still have no faith?'
>
> The disciples were absolutely terrified. 'Who is this man?' they asked each other. 'Even the wind and waves obey him!'"

I love that Jesus was sleeping at the back of the boat because that is where the stern, or the wheel, is located in boats and ships. This is where the captain steers and controls the direction. Reread Mark 4:35. Jesus says, "Let's cross to the other side of the lake." They were going to make it to the other side no matter what because Christ said it. Today we live in a society with a go-go-go, run-run-run mindset. This way of thinking never allows us to slow down, rest, reflect, or simply enjoy life. We feel we are going to miss something great that next bonus, that next big opportunity, that next life changing phone call, etc. We have fed our minds the lie of, "we will not make it to the other side of the lake." Because we believe this lie, we go-go-go and run-run-run. The truth is our minds, bodies, and spirits need to, and must rest. Some of the best and most rewarding ideas are produced in rest and solitude.

You must know and believe that resting is not going to delay you from crossing to the other side of the lake.

Day 7
Unlocking My Optimal Performance

Moment of Truth: Our minds, body, and spirit need to, and have to have rest.

Verse to Remember: "He makes me lie down in green pastures, he leads me beside quiet waters."
Psalms 23:2 (NIV)

Challenge to Implement: Identify and implement one way you can give up the go-go-go run-run-run mentality and simply rest more.

Soli Deo Gloria and Arise!®

Candice

Day 7 - Sleep to Live

Sleep profoundly affects our quality of life. Sadly, we are oblivious to our diminished capabilities because we have become a society conditioned to function on low levels of alertness. Some people no longer know what it feels like to be fully awake anymore. Sleep should not be taken for granted. In fact, think how much more effective we could be with optimal sleep. Sleep prepares our mind and body for optimal performance. Quality sleep restores, rejuvenates, and energizes our body and brain.

Sleep Effects

Alertness	Energy
Mood	Bodyweight
Perception	Memory/Thinking
Reaction Time	Productivity
Performance	Communication Skills
Creativity	Safety
Health	Exercise Intensity
Restoration & Growth of Muscle	Immunity to Viral Infections

Unfortunately, in today's hectic society we no longer value sleep. People who sleep six hours or less are considered tough, competitive, and ambitious. If you say you need lots of sleep, some perceive you as one who lacks what it takes to be successful. Consequently, half of the adult population is studying, working, parenting, or driving while exhausted. As a result, we make costly mental errors and are more accident-prone. We become sick far too easily, and often. We have become a world at risk because we do not understand the need for sleep or the consequences of sleep deprivation. We must learn to value sleep as much as we value the importance of proper nutrition and exercise. To unlock optimal performance, we must change our habits.

Once you value sleep and understand your individual sleep requirement, you can improve your sleep quality. Adopting sound sleep habits is imperative to overall fitness. A better night's sleep improves your energy, efficiency, and it makes you feel better overall. Many people who improve their sleep improve their waking lives because they are more present and aware of their spouses, their children, and their careers. What kind of life do you want to live?

What Sleep Accomplishes

Assists Physical Recovery	Improves Retention
Promotes Tissue Growth and Repair	Improves Memory Retention
Heightened Alertness	Better Memory Recall
Higher Energy Levels	Better Memory Organization
Improved Overall Health	Strengthens Immunity Against Viral Infections

Day 7
Unlocking My Optimal Performance

Moment of Truth: Often we are completely unaware of our own reduced capabilities because we have become habituated to low levels of alertness.

Quote to Remember: "The body needs its rest, and sleep is extremely important in any health regimen. There should be three main things: eating, exercise and sleep. All three together in the right balance make for a truly healthy lifestyle."
- Rohit Shetty

Challenge to Implement: List two ways sleep has affected your quality of life.

Soli Deo Gloria and *Arise!*®

Candice

Two ways sleep has affected my quality of life:

1)

2)

Week 2

Day 8

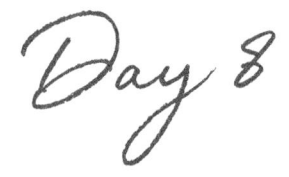

Calorie Counting is Inexact

As mentioned in Day 1, one of my go-to inspirational scriptures is Jeremiah 29:11.

> "For I know the plans I have for you," says the Lord. "They are plans for good and not for disaster, to give you a future and a hope."

There are many times in life when God sends us small warnings that we choose to ignore. As our Father, I wonder how many times He holds his breath and grimaces, watching us ignore them. Then I wonder how often His heart aches with knowing He must send us additional warnings that become increasingly severe. First it is a speed bump, then a yield sign, next a stop sign, followed by a stop light. Having failed to listen or respond to any of these signals, we pridefully continue down the same road. The next warning sign is a roadblock, but we figure this cannot be right. We then inch our way through the roadblock because we figure a little off-road driving will not hurt. Wrong! Finally, God has to simply take out the bridge we are approaching because this is the only way to prevent us from traveling along the wrong road.

It seems ridiculous that we continue to miss sign after sign. Still, this is what many of us often do; we do not stop to listen, rest, pray, fellowship, etc. How we get from Point A to Point B is an inexact path, but the great news is that we will arrive at Point B because God knows His plans for us.

Day 8
Unlocking My Optimal Performance

Moment of Truth: Many times in life God gives us and sends us small warning signs that we often choose to ignore.

Verse to Remember: *"For I know the plans I have for you," says the Lord. "They are plans for good and not for disaster, to give you a future and a hope."*

Jeremiah 29:11 (NLT)

Challenge to Implement: *Think about the warning signs you have missed in the past. How has this delayed you from getting to Point B?*

Soli Deo Gloria and *Arise!*®

Candice

When was the last time you counted and kept track of all the calories you ate? How long did you do this for? How frustrated did you become with this time consuming task? I have good news for you. Stop calorie counting! It is a waste of time and with today's fast paced society, no one has time to waste. Remember Day 5's lesson: It is all about energy balance and keeping things simple. If you are going for weight loss, consume less calories than you expend. Focus on simply eating clean.

Tomorrow, we will dive into portion sizes. For those who need scientific evidence, here are three reasons why you are wasting your time calorie counting:

Day 8 - Calorie Counting is Inexact

1. Energy is lost through the digestion process. Only about 91% of the energy present in the food we eat can be used for energy transfer.

2. The macronutrients and calorie values contained on food labels are mere approximations. Their measurements are not exact.

3. Our digestion and excretion rates affect the amount of potential energy available once the food is eaten. Since digestion and absorption can vary from 2-5%, and excretion can vary even more, even if you know the exact calorie content of the food you eat, you could not know exactly how much of that energy would become usable energy.

Nutrition Facts

Serving Size 1 egg (50g)

Amount Per Serving	
Calories 70	Calories from Fat 40
	% Daily Value*
Total Fat 3g	7%
Sat. Fat 1.5g	8%
Trans Fat 0g	
Cholest. 215mg	71%
Sodium 65mg	3%
Total Carb. Less than 1g	0%
Protein 6g	10%

Vitamin A	6%	Vitamin C	0%
Calcium	2%	Iron	4%

Not a significant source of Dietary Fiber or Sugars.

If you try your best to approximate your calorie intake, you could be off by anywhere from 8-10%, or more. Adding more variability is the fact that you would be trying to balance this intake with some known level of energy expenditure. Energy expenditure is even harder to pin down than intake.

Unless you live in a research lab and can subject both your intake and expenditure to tightly controlled laboratory measures, trying to calorie count is a losing battle. Food labels and energy expenditure equations are just estimations.

Day 8
Unlocking My Optimal Performance

Moment of Truth: Trying to calorie count is a losing battle. Food labels and energy expenditure equations are just estimations, and not very good ones at that.

Quote to Remember: *"Stop calorie counting!"*
— Candice McField

Challenge to Implement: *If you have ever implemented calorie counting, reflect on how long you did it for and record any frustrations you had with calorie counting.*

Soli Deo Gloria and *Arise!*®

Candice

My frustrations with trying to calorie count in the past:

1)

2)

3)

Day 9

Portions - A Needed Sacrifice

Abraham completed one of the greatest acts of obedience recorded in history. In Genesis 22:2 God commands,
> "Take your son, your only son - yes, Isaac, whom you love so much - and go to the land of Moriah. Go and sacrifice him as a burnt offering on one of the mountains, which I will show you."

Abraham immediately responds to God by getting up the next morning and going to sacrifice his son. Wow! No words can describe that level of obedience. I do not have kids, but I do have a niece and nephew whom I would protect at all costs. Thankfully, Abraham was not like most of us and stood the test of God's refining hand. He was willing to make the ultimate sacrifice, giving up the thing he loved most, all to demonstrate his commitment to obey God. Plus, he deepened his understanding of how God's timing is always perfect.

I love how Paul explains in Philippians 4:11-13,
> "I have learned how to be content with whatever I have. I know how to live on almost nothing or with everything. I have learned the secret of living in every situation, whether it is with a full stomach or empty, with plenty or little. For I can do everything through Christ, who gives me strength."

In our lives, we must make sacrifices to achieve our desired results. Whether it is portion control to drop a few pounds, or obtaining higher education to land our dream job, nothing great comes easy or without sacrifice. The goal is to be content through all the peaks and valleys of life.

Day 7
Unlocking My Optimal Performance

Moment of Truth: We must make sacrifices to achieve our desired results.

Verse to Remember: *"Take your son, your only son - yes, Isaac, whom you love so much - and go to the land of Moriah. Go and sacrifice him as a burnt offering on one of the mountains, which I will show you."*

Genesis 22:2 (NLT)

Challenge to Implement: *Take action towards a life goal you have not achieved yet and begin making a sacrifice to complete that goal.*

Soli Deo Gloria and *Arise!*®

Candice

Over the last twenty years we have made drastic increases to our portion sizes. For example, twenty years ago a bagel was 3-inches in diameter and 140 calories. Now, a bagel is 6-inches in diameter and 350 calories. Twenty years ago, a soda was 6.5 ounces and 85 calories. Today, a soda is 20 ounces and 300 calories. Consequently, increases in portion sizes directly contribute to our growing obesity epidemic, worldwide.

What is the difference between a portion and a serving?

Day 9 - Portions - A Needed Sacrifice

A portion is the amount of food a person <u>chooses</u> to eat. A serving is a standardized amount of a food used to estimate intake.

For most, estimating the portion size they need is very difficult which could mean the difference between a 1,400-calorie and 2,200-calorie diet. To make matters worse, we learned in Day 8 that calorie counting is a waste of time. Therefore, a quick, easy, and reliable way to estimate portion sizes is needed. I believe in, teach, and recommend you use the visual method. Comparing food portions to common items is a quick, helpful way to visualize the foods you eat, adopt better habits, and eat more appropriate food amounts.

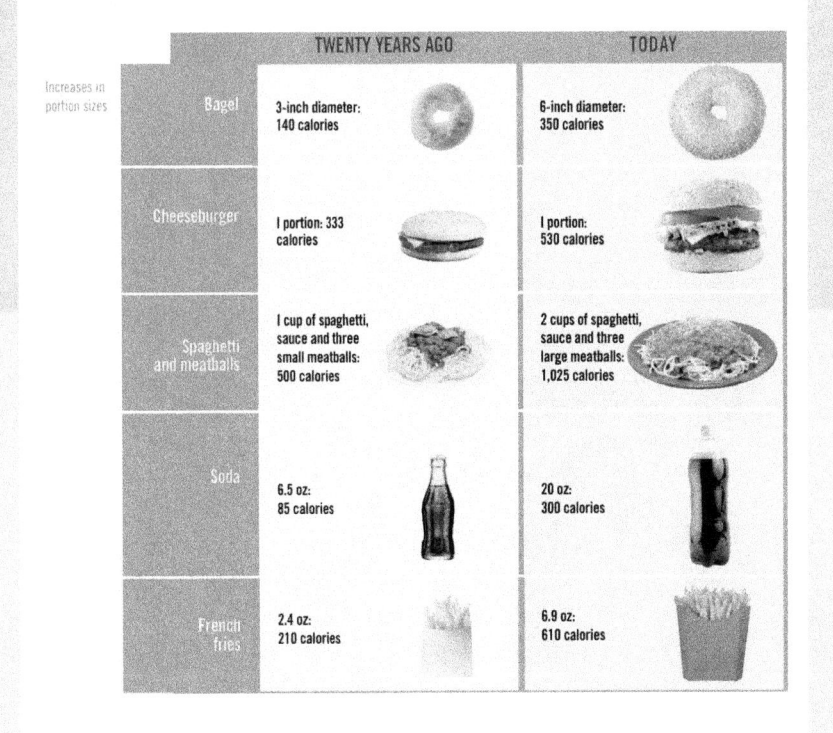

Increases in portion sizes		TWENTY YEARS AGO	TODAY
	Bagel	3-inch diameter: 140 calories	6-inch diameter: 350 calories
	Cheeseburger	1 portion: 333 calories	1 portion: 530 calories
	Spaghetti and meatballs	1 cup of spaghetti, sauce and three small meatballs: 500 calories	2 cups of spaghetti, sauce and three large meatballs: 1,025 calories
	Soda	6.5 oz: 85 calories	20 oz: 300 calories
	French fries	2.4 oz: 210 calories	6.9 oz: 610 calories

Estimating Portion Sizes

Food Group	Visual Portion Size
Protein	Meats = Palm of your hand (men: 2 palms) Peanut butter = ½ Golf ball Nuts = ½ post it note
Grains	Baseball
Fruit	Fresh fruit = Baseball Dried fruit = 2 Golf balls
Vegetables	Softball
Dairy	Milk, Yogurts = Baseball Cheese = 1.5 Nine volt batteries
Oils	Tip of thumb

Day 9
Unlocking My Optimal Performance

Moment of Truth: Increases in portion sizes directly contribute to our growing worldwide obesity epidemic.

Quote to Remember: "I've always practiced this: Love yourself. Move your body. Watch your portions."
— Richard Simmons

Challenge to Implement: List the 10 foods you eat most often. Then, fill in their corresponding visual portion size.

Soli Deo Gloria and *Arise!*®

Candice

Day 1 - Portions - A Needed Sacrifice

My Visual Portion Sizes

My 10 Most Common Foods	Visual Portion Size
1)	
2)	
3)	
4)	
5)	
6)	
7)	
8)	
9)	
10)	

Day 10

Ninety Percent Accuracy

In life we are called to always put our best effort forward. In 2003, I was at Semester at Sea, a study abroad program, touring Japan. I went to Hiroshima and our tour guide told us a Japanese phrase that I loved from the moment I heard it and have never forgotten it. *Ichigo~Ichie*. In fact, it has become my life motto and I even rock it as a tattoo.

Ichigo-Ichie can be translated as "one encounter, one chance" or one life, one chance. It is a long used Japanese phrase that refers to the concept that each instant or encounter is the first, the one, and the only of its kind, never to be repeated. With Ichigo-Ichie, the implication is that our behavior in a given moment has significant, if not lasting, impact upon our lives and the lives of others. Applying the concept of Ichigo-Ichie means to put our best heart forward in every encounter. I summarize Ichigo-Ichie as; one life, one chance - thus make every moment count.

Likewise, in Ephesians 5:16, Paul states, *"Make the most of every opportunity in these evil days."* Then in Colossians 4:5, he commands, *"Live wisely among those who are not believers, and make the most of every opportunity."*

We will never reach perfection, but we can strive to be our best, do our best, and always put our best foot forward.

As For Me and My Body

Day 10
Unlocking My Optimal Performance

Moment of Truth: We will never reach perfection, but we can strive to be our best, do our best, and always put our best foot forward.

Verse to Remember: "Make the most of every opportunity in these evil days."

Ephesians 5:16 (NLT)

Challenge to Implement: Think of one area in which you are not putting your best heart forward. Then implement one solution to do better.

Soli Deo Gloria and *Arise!*®

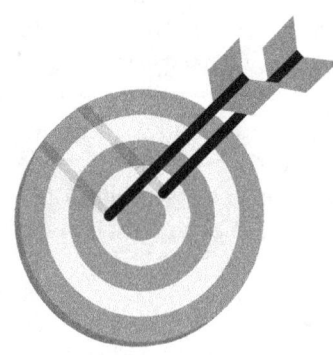

Candice

There is a saying, "To wait for perfection is to wait forever!" The same thing is true for your health and fitness goals. If you aim for 100% accuracy all the time with your health and fitness goals, you will find yourself waiting forever to achieve perfect results. Instead, I recommend striving for 85 to 100% accuracy, depending on which 'training season' you are in. I teach my clients that you cannot stay in a high-intense 100% effort mode forever. This creates burnout.

Think of an athlete. Athletes do not and cannot stay in

Day 10 - Ninety Percent Accuracy

high-intensity training modes forever. Neither can you. Besides burnout, prolonged periods of high intensity training, causes you to be more susceptible to injury. To prevent this, one should stay in a high-intensity training mode for 4 to 6 weeks only. During these 4 to 6 weeks, you are striving for 100% accuracy with every aspect of your training, nutrition, sleep and overall health regimen.

On the opposite end of being in a high-intensity training mode, there are also times when you need to rest your body. In fact, resting your body is a necessity. For instance, if you were in a high intensity training mode for the last 6 weeks to obtain whatever goal you set for yourself, it is now time to roll into a low to medium intensity training period for various intervals. It is critical to give your body built in breaks. This does not mean you stop working out and completely blow your nutrition. Rather, you are now aiming for less than 100% accuracy with your training, nutrition, sleep and overall health regimen.

You do not stay in a low-intensity training mode for the rest of the year either. I recommend fluctuating between 85 and 95% accuracy and striving for 90% accuracy, 90% of the time. The key is to listen to your body and evaluate when and what you want to achieve next. This will determine what level of accuracy you need to strive for and when you need to ramp up from 85%.

Part of this is knowing your body and what works for you, which is why listening and understanding your body is crucial. Some people may be able to strive for 85% accuracy to maintain their physique while for some they will have to be higher than 85%.

I believe in keeping things simple. A good rule to follow is:
- 90% of your training duration, strive for 90% accuracy
- 5% of your training duration, strive for 100% accuracy
- 5% of your training duration, strive for 85% accuracy

CMF Training Guidelines

Duration	Accuracy Level	Training Intensities
90% of the time	90%	Moderate to Medium
5% of the time	100%	High
5% of the time	85%	Low

	90% Accuracy Examples
Nutrition	If you are eating 5 meals per day. That is 35 meals per week. 90% accuracy equates 3 cheat meals per week. (10% of 35, rounded down)
Exercise	If you are working out 5 days per week. That is 20 workouts per month. 90% accuracy equates 2 missed workout sessions per month. (10% of 20)
Sleep	If you are sleeping 7 hours per night. That is 49 hours of sleep per week. 90% accuracy equates 5 hours of missed sleep for the week. (10% of 49, rounded up)

Day 10

Unlocking My Optimal Performance

Moment of Truth: If you aim for 100% accuracy all the time with your health and fitness goals, you will find yourself waiting forever to achieve perfect results.

Quote to Remember: *"Perfection is not attainable, but if we chase perfection we can catch excellence."*
— Vince Lombardi

Challenge to Implement: Calculate what you must do to achieve 90% accuracy in each critical area: nutrition, workout sessions, and sleep.

Soli Deo Gloria and *Arise!*®

Candice

To achieve 90% accuracy:

I can have _____ cheat meals per week.

I can miss _____ workout sessions per week.

I can miss _____ hours of sleep _____ per week.

Day 11

Mature with Strength Training

In our Christian walk, we are called to constantly grow and mature in our walk with Christ. Possessing unshakable faith is one of those steps towards maturing in our walk. While rereading the gospels one summer, I discovered how Jesus took particular notice of those with unshakable faith, healing and cherishing them. One of the best stories displaying unshakable faith is that of the Roman officer found in Mathew 8:6-13.

> "Lord, my young servant lies in bed, paralyzed and in terrible pain." Jesus said, 'I will come and heal him.' But the officer said, "Lord, I am not worthy to have you come into my home. Just say the word from where you are, and my servant will be healed. I know this because I am under the authority of my superior officers, and I have authority over my soldiers. I only need to say, 'Go,' and they go, or 'Come,' and they come. And if I say to my slaves, 'Do this,' they do it." When Jesus heard this, he was amazed. Turning to those who were following him, he said, 'I tell you the truth, I haven't seen faith like this in all Israel!'... Then Jesus said to the Roman officer, 'Go back home. Because you believed, it has happened.' And the young servant was healed that same hour."

For all exercise programs, you must mature with your regimen by adding in strength training. There are many people who focus only on cardio and wonder why they lack definition. In order to shape and define muscles, you must strength train.

Day 11
Unlocking My Optimal Performance

Moment of Truth: Jesus took notice of, healed, and cherished those with unshakable faith.

Verse to Remember: "Then Jesus said to the Roman officer, 'Go back home. Because you believed, it has happened.' And the young servant was healed the same hour."
                                                                Matthew 8:13 (NLT)

Challenge to Implement: What area of your life do you need to have more faith with or in? Turn this area completely over to God. Completely, surrendering control to Him equates to an unexplainable freedom and blessing.

Soli Deo Gloria and *Arise!*®

Candice

Have you ever heard of the term "skinny fat?" It refers to someone who "looks" skinny but actually has a higher percentage of body fat than desired. They may look good in clothes but that is it. Unfortunately, many people fall into the skinny fat category because they do not or have never made strength training part of their workout regimen. If you do not strength train, you will simply become a smaller version of your bigger self! Strength training is critical to unlocking optimal performance because it shapes and defines your body's composition, increases your metabolic function, and it reduces your risk of injury.

Day 11 - Mature with Strength Training

Body composition refers to the makeup of total body mass, which is divided into two types of mass: fat-free and fat. Fat-free mass is composed of bone, muscle, and organs while fat mass is composed of connective tissue, made up of fat cells.

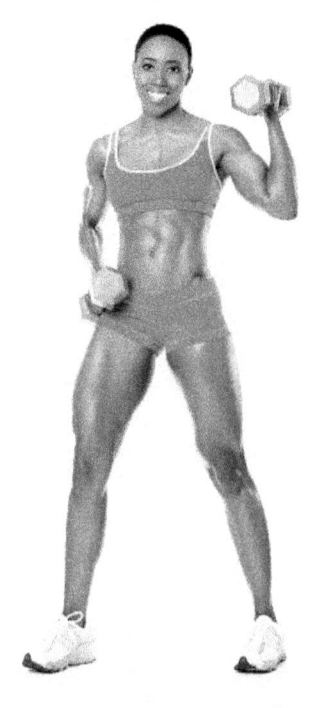

Unfortunately, ideal body weight has historically been determined without concern for body composition and involved the use of the standardized height-weight tables, such as the tables used in body mass index (BMI) calculations. Ideal body weight is estimated only from height and weight without consideration of the composition of the weight. Therefore, a well-conditioned bodybuilder might be considered overweight based on height and weight. Meanwhile, another person could fall within the accepted range but be fat by body composition standards.

It is not uncommon for an exerciser to lose pounds of fat and gain pounds of muscle without any change in total body weight. Therefore, you should always remember muscle is heavier than fat. Consider a 130-pound woman who has 24% body fat. Of her total body weight, 31 of those pounds are from fat mass and 99 of those pounds are from fat-free mass. If she loses 4 pounds of fat and adds 4 pounds of muscle she will still weigh 130 pounds but will have only 20% body fat. Her 31 pounds of fat mass drops to 27 and her fat-free mass increases from 99 to 103. Although her body weight remains the same, she has less fat and more muscle for a leaner, firmer, and more fit appearance.

To track your progress, I recommend you use the following, instead of BMI: circumference measurements, waist-to-hip ratio, percentage of body fat, changes in clothes sizes, energy levels, overall attitude, and weight.

Strength Training Facts

1. Muscles are responsible for more than 25% of our calorie use.

2. An increase in muscle tissue causes a corresponding increase in our metabolic rate.
   - The higher the metabolic rate = higher metabolism = higher calories burned.

3. We lose more than ½ of a pound of muscle every year of life after age 25.
   - This leads to a 5% reduction in metabolic rate every decade unless we strength train.
   - This gradual decrease in metabolism is closely related to the gradual increase in body fat that typically accompanies the aging process.
   - Calories previously used by muscle tissue get stored as fat.

4. Although our metabolism eventually slows down with age, this, and other degenerative processes, such as, heart disease, diabetes, and osteoporosis can be delayed through regular strength training.

5. Muscles serve as shock absorbers and balancing agents.

6. Balanced muscle development reduces the risk of overuse injuries.

7. Four out of five Americans experience lower back discomfort. However, 80% of lower back problems are muscular in nature and appear to be preventable by strengthening the lower back muscles.

Day 11
Unlocking My Optimal Performance

Moment of Truth: If you do not strength train, you will simply become a skinnier version of your bigger self!

Quote to Remember: *"Not lifting weights because you are afraid of looking like a bodybuilder is like not driving your car because you fear becoming a NASCAR driver."*
- Anonymous

Challenge to Implement: Pick at least four out of the six progress measures to track your health and fitness journey. Record where you are today.

Soli Deo Gloria and *Arise!*®

Candice

Circumference Measurements

Bicep:	**Hips:**
Take the measurement half way between the shoulder and elbow at the maximum girth of your bicep.	Take measurement at the maximal girth of your glutes.
Chest:	**Quadricep:**
Take the measurement at the nipple level.	Take the measurement half-way between your hip and knee at the maximal girth of your quad.
Waist:	**Calf:**
Take the measurement at the narrowest part of your waist above your naval. It is where you have a natural bend in the waist.	Take the measurement at the maximum girth between your knee and ankle.
Abdomen:	Notes:
Take the tape measurement at your navel level.	

Waist-to-Hip Ratio

Divide your waist measurement by your hip measurement.

My Waist/Hip is:	My Classification is:

Classification	Women	Men
High Risk	> 0.85	> 1.0
Moderately High Risk	0.80 - 0.85	0.90 - 1.0
Lower Risk	< 0.80	< 0.90

Day 11 - Mature with Strength Training

Percentage of Bodyfat for Women

My bodyfat percentage is:

Age	20 - 30	30 - 40	40 - 50	50+
Very Low Fat	< 17%	< 18%	< 20%	< 21%
Low Fat	17 - 20%	18 - 21%	20 - 23%	21 - 24%
Average Fat	21 - 23 %	23 - 25%	24 - 27%	26 - 28%
Very High Fat	24 - 27%	25 - 29%	28 - 31%	31 - 35%
Overfat	28+	30+	32+	36+

Percentage of Bodyfat for Men

My bodyfat percentage is:

Age	20 - 30	30 - 40	40 - 50	50+
Very Low Fat	< 9%	< 11%	< 12%	< 13%
Low Fat	9 - 12%	11 - 13%	12 - 15%	13 - 16%
Average Fat	13 - 16%	14 - 17%	16 - 20%	17 - 21%
Very High Fat	17 - 19%	18 - 22%	21 - 25%	22 - 27%
Overfat	20+	23+	26+	28+

Clothes Sizes

Shirt:	Pants:	Dress:

Energy Levels
Circle one

Compared to my peers, I have:

More , The Same, or Less Energy

As For Me and My Body

Attitude
Honestly evaluate your attitude over the last 11 days

Over the last 11 days, my attitude has been

_____
_____
_____
_____
_____

Weight

My weight today is:

Day 12

Muscle Groups Unify

On Day 4, I stated how Thunderbird was always my dream school. I decided to fulfill my dream of attending Thunderbird all in a matter of four weeks. It was a crazy, scary, and very exciting time in my life. I often look for three confirmations when I am faced with big, life changing decisions which I share on Day 14. For now, I will share a story to illustrate one of the signals, through circumstances.

While fasting and praying over whether I should attend Thunderbird, a dear church member pulled me out of service and into the foyer. She prayed for me and gave me a ring of a Thunderbird. She told me, "I received this ring in 1974 or 1975 from a woman on a Navajo reservation I visited. It was a huge deal for her to take it off her hand and give it to a 'white' person. Clearly, God was at work." I walked back into the church service and scribbled these thoughts on a piece of paper in my Bible, "I'm speechless and humbled beyond imagination of how good God is and how the love of Koinonia Bible Church is so genuine and pure. My heart is touched beyond which words can express from my friend's prayer and gift. I'm trying not to cry. Clearly this is another sign of how I'm supposed to go to Thunderbird and how He is going to make the way. Lord, I cannot thank you enough for my dear friend showing the love of Christ. Please bless her continuously and abundantly." I still have the ring to this day.

What a monumental race relations moment in 1974 between the Native American lady and my friend. Regardless of our faith and beliefs, we must mature in our walk to display love that extends beyond ethnicity and social class. If you read and study Nicodemus in the Book of John, chapters 3, 7, and 19, you see how he matured to the point where he risked his reputation for Jesus and displayed love, despite his privileged social standing as a religious leader.

> *"Then Nicodemus, the leader who had met with Jesus earlier, spoke up. 'Is it legal to convict a man before he is given a hearing?' he asked. They replied, 'Are you from Galilee, too? Search the Scriptures and see for yourself-- no prophet ever comes from Galilee!"* (John 7:50-52)

> *"With him came Nicodemus, the man who had come to Jesus at night. He brought seventy--five pounds of perfumed ointment made from myrrh and aloes. Following Jewish burial custom, they wrapped Jesus' body with the spices in long sheets of linen cloth."* (John 19:39-40)

Let us be inspired by Nicodemus. Show, and give love daily because "everyone smiles in the same language," meaning we are all one unified body of Christ.

While strength training is required to shape and define your body, consistently training each muscle group creates balance and symmetry for your physique. Each major muscle group works together to make a stronger unified body.

Day 12 - Muscle Groups Unify

Day 12
Unlocking My Optimal Performance

Moment of Truth: Regardless of our faith and beliefs, we must mature in our walk to display love that extends beyond ethnicity and social class.

Verse to Remember: *"The human body has many parts, but the many parts make up one whole body. So it is with the body of Christ. Some of us are Jews, some are Gentiles, some are slaves, and some are free. But we have all been baptized into one body by one Spirit, and we all share the same Spirit."*
1 Corinthians 12:12-13 (NLT)

Challenge to Implement: *Perform a random act of kindness for someone that is not in your social, economic, ethnic, or nationality circle.*

Soli Deo Gloria and *Arise!*®

Candice

There are many ways to develop muscle strength. Unfortunately, many strength training programs have a high rate of injury and a low rate of muscle development. The goal is to have safe, effective, and efficient strength training sessions.

It is important to select at least one exercise for each major muscle group to ensure comprehensive muscle development. Training only a few muscle groups leads to muscle imbalance and increases the risk of injury. Fellas, no offense, but one thing I hate to see in the gym are men who only work their upper body. They end up having a developed upper body, a nice V-taper, and chicken legs. For ladies, it is the opposite. Many women focus on developing only their glutes and abs yet lack the upper body development to do one push-up or pull-up. For overall balance, train each major muscle group, at least once, on a weekly basis.

Major Muscle Groups

Biceps	Triceps
Chest	Shoulders
Back	Quadriceps
Hamstrings	Calves
Glutes	Core

The following pages contain total body workouts in which each muscle group is trained. Enjoy!

Day 12 - Muscle Groups Unify

TOTAL BODY
Candice McField Fitness

| 2 sets per exercise | 60 seconds per set | 60 seconds rest between sets |

Equipment: Bodyweight

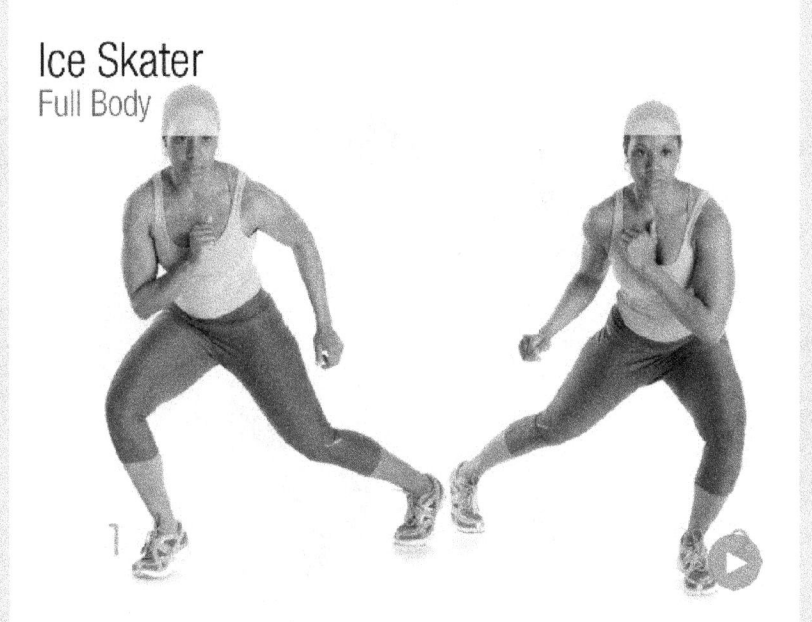

Ice Skater
Full Body

1. Start in a semi-squat position with one leg stretched out to the side.
2. Push off your front leg to jump to the other side, switching your other leg out to the side.
- Use your arms in a swinging motion
- Alternate sides with each rep.

scan the code to view a video of the workout

#	REPS	WEIGHT	TIME	NOTES
1			60.0	
2			60.0	

© 2020. Candice McField Fitness, LLC. All rights reserved. No part of this publication may be reproduced, distributed, or transmitted in any form, without prior written permission of Candice McField Fitness, LLC. User represents that he/she has consulted with a Physician regarding User's potential use of this workout, prior to beginning the workout, and that the physician consents to User's performance of the workout. The content of the workout and any information otherwise obtained by user through the workout is provided for information purposes only and User uses such information and content AT THE VOLUNTARY, SOLE RISK OF THE USER. USER RELEASES AND RELIEVES, AND AGREES TO RELEASE AND RELIEVE, CANDICE MCFIELD FITNESS, LLC. AND LAUNCHCRATE PUBLISHING, LLC. OF ANY AND ALL LIABILITY FOR ANY INJURIES, CLAIMS OR DAMAGES ARISING OUT OF USER'S USE OF THE SERVICE.

TOTAL BODY
Candice McField Fitness

2 sets per exercise **60 seconds** per set **60 seconds** rest between sets

Equipment: Bodyweight, Dumbbells

Kickback
Triceps

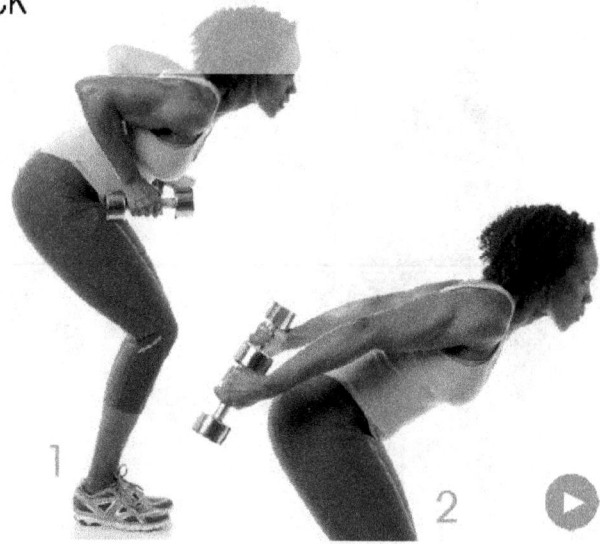

scan the code to view a video of the workout

1. Bend forward 45-degrees from the waist. Hold the dumbbells by your sides and bend your elbows.
2. Lift the dumbbells back, straightening your arms. Keep your elbows still, shoulders steady and your back flat throughout.
- Return to the start position and repeat.

#	REPS	WEIGHT	TIME	NOTES
1			60.0	
2			60.0	

© 2020. Candice McField Fitness, LLC. All rights reserved. No part of this publication may be reproduced, distributed, or transmitted in any form, without prior written permission of Candice McField Fitness, LLC. User represents that he/she has consulted with a Physician regarding User's potential use of this workout, prior to beginning the workout, and that the physician consents to User's performance of the workout. The content of the workout and any information otherwise obtained by user through the workout is provided for information purposes only and User uses such information and content AT THE VOLUNTARY, SOLE RISK OF THE USER. USER RELEASES AND RELIEVES, AND AGREES TO RELEASE AND RELIEVE, CANDICE MCFIELD FITNESS, LLC. AND LAUNCHCRATE PUBLISHING, LLC. OF ANY AND ALL LIABILITY FOR ANY INJURIES, CLAIMS OR DAMAGES ARISING OUT OF USER'S USE OF THE SERVICE.

Day 12 - Muscle Groups Unify

TOTAL BODY
Candice McField Fitness

2 sets	60 seconds	60 seconds
per exercise	per set	rest between sets

Equipment: Bodyweight, Dumbbells

Alternating Press
Shoulders

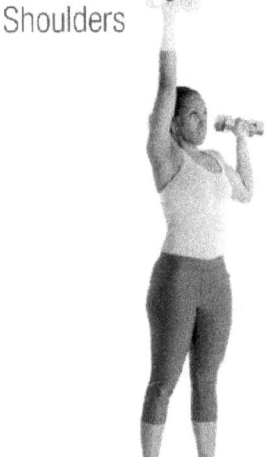

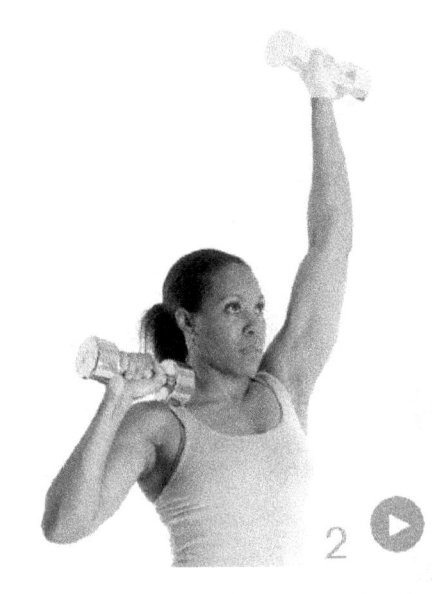

- Stand holding a pair of dumbbells at shoulder height with your elbows bent, palms facing forward.
1. Press one dumbbell overhead, fully extending your arm.
2. Lower the dumbbell, then press the other overhead as you remain upright throughout the movement.
- Alternate sides with each rep.

scan the code to view a video of the workout

#	REPS	WEIGHT	TIME	NOTES
1			60.0	
2			60.0	

© 2020. Candice McField Fitness, LLC. All rights reserved. No part of this publication may be reproduced, distributed, or transmitted in any form, without prior written permission of Candice McField Fitness, LLC. User represents that he/she has consulted with a Physician regarding User's potential use of this workout, prior to beginning the workout, and that the physician consents to User's performance of the workout. The content of the workout and any information otherwise obtained by user through the workout is provided for information purposes only and User uses such information and content AT THE VOLUNTARY, SOLE RISK OF THE USER. USER RELEASES AND RELIEVES, AND AGREES TO RELEASE AND RELIEVE, CANDICE MCFIELD FITNESS, LLC. AND LAUNCHCRATE PUBLISHING, LLC. OF ANY AND ALL LIABILITY FOR ANY INJURIES, CLAIMS OR DAMAGES ARISING OUT OF USER'S USE OF THE SERVICE.

TOTAL BODY
Candice McField Fitness

2 sets per exercise | **60 seconds** per set | **60 seconds** rest between sets

Equipment: Bodyweight, Dumbbells

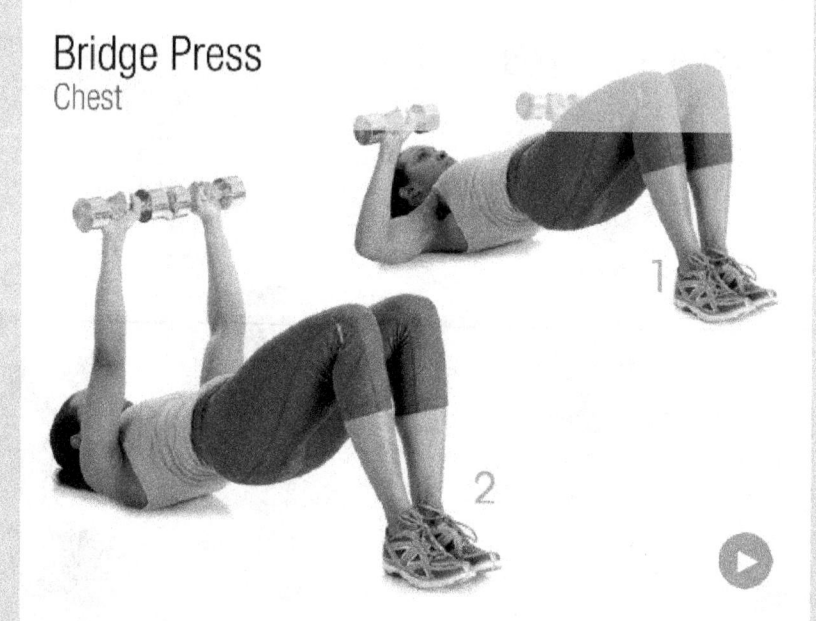

Bridge Press
Chest

- Lie on your back with your knees bent and feet flat. Hold dumbbells at your shoulders with your upper arms on the floor, elbows bent.
1. Raise your hips off the floor and try to make a straight line from your hips to your shoulders.
2. Press the dumbbells up over your chest, extending your arms.
- Lower the dumbbells and repeat.

scan the code to view a video of the workout

#	REPS	WEIGHT	TIME	NOTES
1			60.0	
2			60.0	

© 2020. Candice McField Fitness, LLC. All rights reserved. No part of this publication may be reproduced, distributed, or transmitted in any form, without prior written permission of Candice McField Fitness, LLC. User represents that he/she has consulted with a Physician regarding User's potential use of this workout, prior to beginning the workout, and that the physician consents to User's performance of the workout. The content of the workout and any information otherwise obtained by user through the workout is provided for information purposes only and User uses such information and content AT THE VOLUNTARY, SOLE RISK OF THE USER. USER RELEASES AND RELIEVES, AND AGREES TO RELEASE AND RELIEVE, CANDICE MCFIELD FITNESS, LLC. AND LAUNCHCRATE PUBLISHING, LLC. OF ANY AND ALL LIABILITY FOR ANY INJURIES, CLAIMS OR DAMAGES ARISING OUT OF USER'S USE OF THE SERVICE.

Day 12 - Muscle Groups Unify

TOTAL BODY
Candice McField Fitness

2 sets	60 seconds	60 seconds
per exercise	per set	rest between sets

Equipment: Bodyweight, Dumbbells

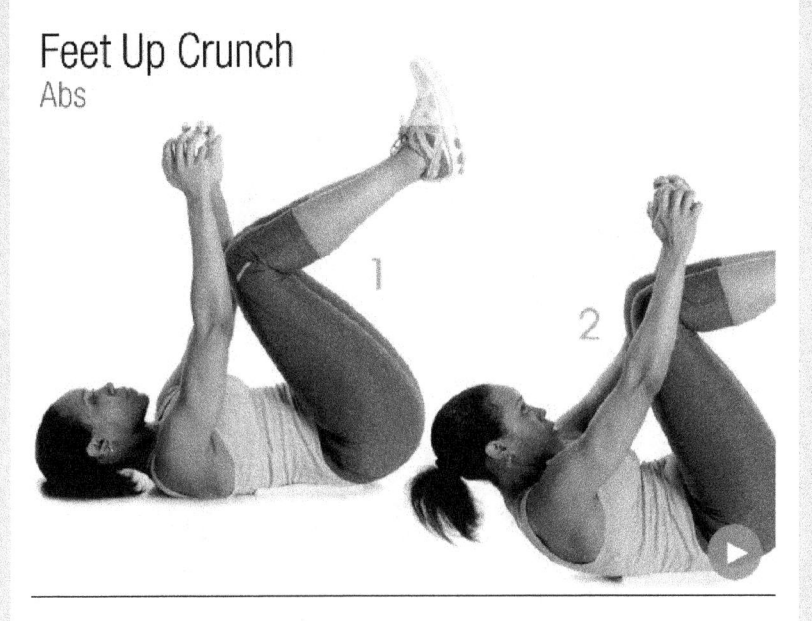

Feet Up Crunch
Abs

1. Lie on your back with your knees bent and feet raised. Hold a dumbbell straight over your chest.
2. Lift your head and shoulders off the floor, keeping your feet raised and arms straight.
- Lower your head and shoulders then repeat.

scan the code to view a video of the workout

#	REPS	WEIGHT	TIME	NOTES
1			60.0	
2			60.0	

© 2020. Candice McField Fitness, LLC. All rights reserved. No part of this publication may be reproduced, distributed, or transmitted in any form, without prior written permission of Candice McField Fitness, LLC. User represents that he/she has consulted with a Physician regarding User's potential use of this workout, prior to beginning the workout, and that the physician consents to User's performance of the workout. The content of the workout and any information otherwise obtained by user through the workout is provided for information purposes only and User uses such information and content AT THE VOLUNTARY, SOLE RISK OF THE USER. USER RELEASES AND RELIEVES, AND AGREES TO RELEASE AND RELIEVE, CANDICE MCFIELD FITNESS, LLC. AND LAUNCHCRATE PUBLISHING, LLC. OF ANY AND ALL LIABILITY FOR ANY INJURIES, CLAIMS OR DAMAGES ARISING OUT OF USER'S USE OF THE SERVICE.

As For Me and My Body

TOTAL BODY
Candice McField Fitness

| 2 sets per exercise | 60 seconds per set | 60 seconds rest between sets |

Equipment: Bodyweight

Lying Back Squeeze
Back

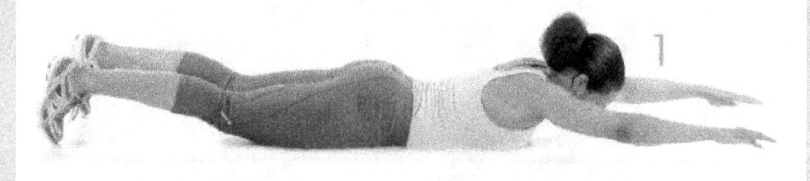

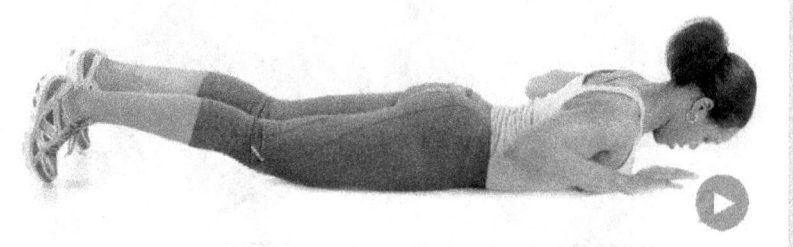

1. Lie face down on the floor with your legs straight and arms overhead.
2. Bend your arms at a 90-degree angle while slowly lowering your arms to your shoulders and squeezing your shoulder blades.
- Hold this position briefly, then return to the start position and repeat.

scan the code to view a video of the workout

#	REPS	WEIGHT	TIME	NOTES
1			60.0	
2			60.0	

© 2020. Candice McField Fitness, LLC. All rights reserved. No part of this publication may be reproduced, distributed, or transmitted in any form, without prior written permission of Candice McField Fitness, LLC. User represents that he/she has consulted with a Physician regarding User's potential use of this workout, prior to beginning the workout, and that the physician consents to User's performance of the workout. The content of the workout and any information otherwise obtained by user through the workout is provided for information purposes only and User uses such information and content AT THE VOLUNTARY, SOLE RISK OF THE USER. USER RELEASES AND RELIEVES, AND AGREES TO RELEASE AND RELIEVE, CANDICE MCFIELD FITNESS, LLC. AND LAUNCHCRATE PUBLISHING, LLC. OF ANY AND ALL LIABILITY FOR ANY INJURIES, CLAIMS OR DAMAGES ARISING OUT OF USER'S USE OF THE SERVICE.

Day 12 - Muscle Groups Unify

TOTAL BODY
Candice McField Fitness

2 sets	60 seconds	60 seconds
per exercise	per set	rest between sets

Equipment: Bodyweight, Dumbbells

Reverse Lunge
Legs

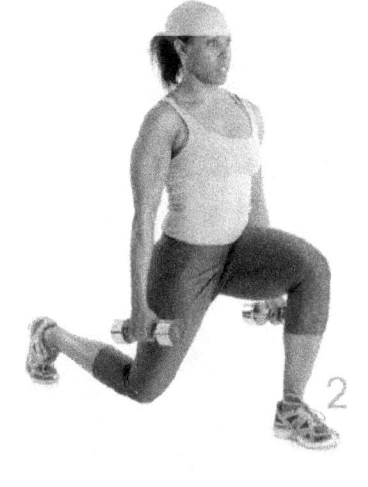

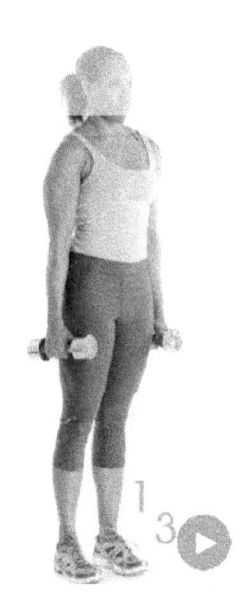

scan the code to view a video of the workout

1. Stand holding dumbbells down by your sides.
2. Take a step backward, drop your back knee to the floor and slightly lean your torso forward, bearing your weight on your front leg.
3. Push off your front heel and return to the start position.
- Complete all reps on one side before switching to the other side.

#	REPS	WEIGHT	TIME	NOTES
1			60.0	
2			60.0	

© 2020. Candice McField Fitness, LLC. All rights reserved. No part of this publication may be reproduced, distributed, or transmitted in any form, without prior written permission of Candice McField Fitness, LLC. User represents that he/she has consulted with a Physician regarding User's potential use of this workout, prior to beginning the workout, and that the physician consents to User's performance of the workout. The content of the workout and any information otherwise obtained by user through the workout is provided for information purposes only and User uses such information and content AT THE VOLUNTARY, SOLE RISK OF THE USER. USER RELEASES AND RELIEVES, AND AGREES TO RELEASE AND RELIEVE, CANDICE MCFIELD FITNESS, LLC. AND LAUNCHCRATE PUBLISHING, LLC. OF ANY AND ALL LIABILITY FOR ANY INJURIES, CLAIMS OR DAMAGES ARISING OUT OF USER'S USE OF THE SERVICE.

TOTAL BODY
Candice McField Fitness

| 2 sets per exercise | 60 seconds per set | 60 seconds rest between sets |

Equipment: Bodyweight, Dumbbells

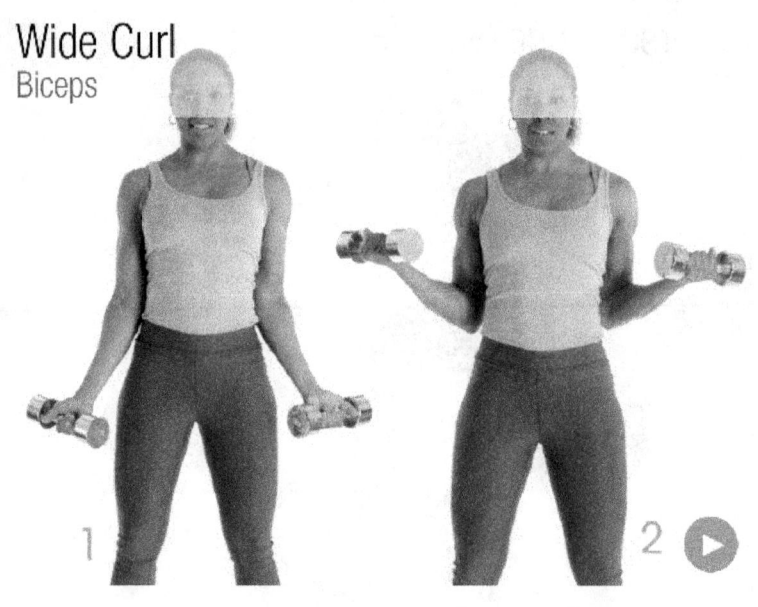

Wide Curl
Biceps

scan the code to view a video of the workout

1. Stand with your arms extended holding dumbbells with your palms facing outward. Externally rotate your shoulders so the dumbbells are at a 45 degree angle from your body.
2. Raise the dumbbells up to shoulder height, bending at the elbows.

#	REPS	WEIGHT	TIME	NOTES
1			60.0	
2			60.0	

© 2020. Candice McField Fitness, LLC. All rights reserved. No part of this publication may be reproduced, distributed, or transmitted in any form, without prior written permission of Candice McField Fitness, LLC. User represents that he/she has consulted with a Physician regarding User's potential use of this workout, prior to beginning the workout, and that the physician consents to User's performance of the workout. The content of the workout and any information otherwise obtained by user through the workout is provided for information purposes only and User uses such information and content AT THE VOLUNTARY, SOLE RISK OF THE USER. USER RELEASES AND RELIEVES, AND AGREES TO RELEASE AND RELIEVE, CANDICE MCFIELD FITNESS, LLC. AND LAUNCHCRATE PUBLISHING, LLC. OF ANY AND ALL LIABILITY FOR ANY INJURIES, CLAIMS OR DAMAGES ARISING OUT OF USER'S USE OF THE SERVICE.

Day 12 - Muscle Groups Unify

TOTAL BODY
Candice McField Fitness

| 2 sets per exercise | 60 seconds per set | 60 seconds rest between sets |

Equipment: Bodyweight

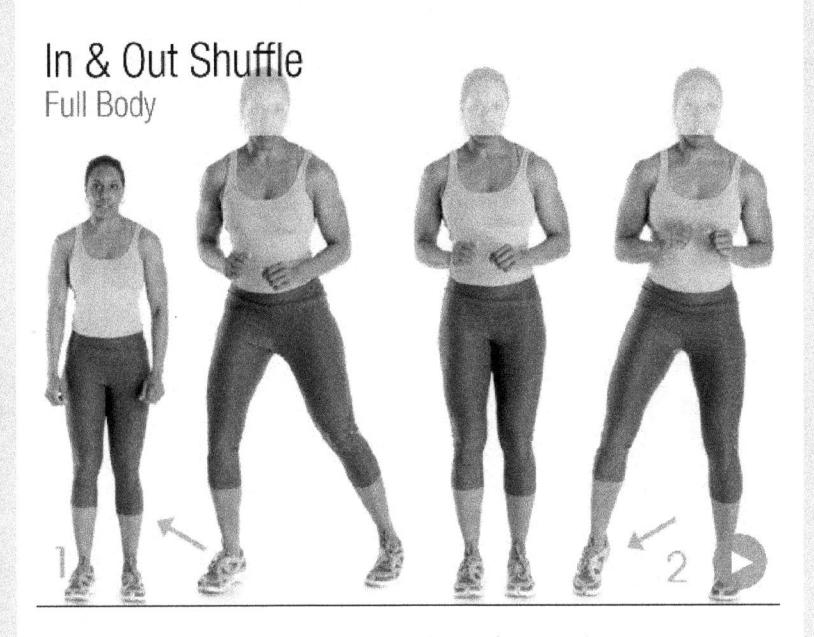

In & Out Shuffle
Full Body

1. Stand upright with your feet together.
2. Rapidly step one foot, then the other foot, 1 to 2 feet in front and to each side.
3. Rapidly step the first foot, then the other foot, back in together to the start position.
- Continue rapidly stepping out in front then back to the start position.

scan the code to view a video of the workout

#	REPS	WEIGHT	TIME	NOTES
1			60.0	
2			60.0	

© 2020. Candice McField Fitness, LLC. All rights reserved. No part of this publication may be reproduced, distributed, or transmitted in any form, without prior written permission of Candice McField Fitness, LLC. User represents that he/she has consulted with a Physician regarding User's potential use of this workout, prior to beginning the workout, and that the physician consents to User's performance of the workout. The content of the workout and any information otherwise obtained by user through the workout is provided for information purposes only and User uses such information and content AT THE VOLUNTARY, SOLE RISK OF THE USER. USER RELEASES AND RELIEVES, AND AGREES TO RELEASE AND RELIEVE, CANDICE MCFIELD FITNESS, LLC. AND LAUNCHCRATE PUBLISHING, LLC. OF ANY AND ALL LIABILITY FOR ANY INJURIES, CLAIMS OR DAMAGES ARISING OUT OF USER'S USE OF THE SERVICE.

As For Me and My Body

Day 12
Unlocking My Optimal Performance

Moment of Truth: Training each major muscle group is critical to ensure comprehensive muscle development.

Quote to Remember: *"It is pointless to have an incredible V- taper with chicken legs!"*

— Candice McField

Challenge to Implement: Name two major muscle groups you fail to consistently train. Add those two muscle groups into to your strength training regimen.

Soli Deo Gloria and *Arise!*®

Candice

Two major muscle groups I fail to consistently train:

1.

2.

Day 13

Cardio - Movement Towards Your Finish Line

I learned so much as a member of Kingdom Advisors when I worked in finance from creating a lifetime gifting goal that affects Kingdom work, to hearing Dr. Tony Evans deliver a keynote speech at the 2006 annual conference which stressed the importance of doing what you do as a calling and not simply as a career. Another Kingdom Advisor takeaway I keep dear to my heart is the phrase, "a sprinter always knows where the finish line is." We should all know what we are striving to achieve. If we do not have a specific marker, human nature will cause us to constantly keep chasing after the next thing. Unless we know *what* and *where* our finish line is, we will never be satisfied with what we have, where we are going, or what we have achieved.

Paul laments in 1 Corinthians 9: 24-27,

> *"Do not you realize that in a race everyone runs, but only one person gets the prize? So run to win! All athletes are disciplined in their training. They do it to win a prize that will fade away, but we do it for an eternal prize. So I run with purpose in every step. I am not just shadowboxing. I discipline my body like an athlete, training it to do what it should do."*

We must have purpose with every step we take in life. For example, when you do cardio, keeping your long-term goal, your finish line (ex. losing 20 pounds) at the forefront of your mind will propel you during the cardio session or on the days you do not necessarily want to do cardio. Spiritually, we go through test and trials that seem impossible to overcome, yet if we keep our eye on the prize, know our finish line, and remember the promises of God we will indeed finish the race.

Day 13
Unlocking My Optimal Performance

Moment of Truth: We must have purpose with every step we take in life.

Verse to Remember: *"So I run with purpose in every step. I am not just shadowboxing."*

1 Corinthians 9:26 (NLT)

Challenge to Implement: *Reflect on and define your finish line for different areas of your life. Possible areas could include: spiritual, relationships, health and fitness, education, and financial.*

Soli Deo Gloria and *Arise!*®

Candice

Day 13 - Cardio - Movement Towards your Finish Line

Having superb cardiovascular health is incredibly important to your overall health and it goes beyond increasing your stamina and endurance. It defines the status of the heart muscle, its blood vessels, and the circulatory system it serves. People with superb cardiovascular health have more stamina, less fatigue, and fewer risks for injury.

Reported Health Benefits of Cardio

Reduction in blood pressure	Decreased anxiety
Increased HDL cholesterol	Decreased tension
Decreased total cholesterol	Decreased depression
Decreased body fat stores	Increased heart function
Increased aerobic work capacity	Prevention of Type II Diabetes

There are two major extremes regarding people doing cardio. First, you have the people who love strength training and hate doing cardio so they never, or hardly ever, do cardio. On the opposite end, you have those that only do cardio. The truth is, you cannot build and maintain an incredible physique without doing both cardio and strength training.

Two frequently asked questions I receive about cardio are:
1. Does low-intensity exercise burn the more fat?
2. Should I work out in the morning, evening or at night?

A very common misconception is that low-intensity exercise is the best way to lose body weight and, more specifically, body fat. It is beyond the scope of this book to prove scientifically, but research proves 30 minutes of low-intensity exercise versus 30 minutes of high intensity exercise results in a lower total number of fat calories burned during the low-intensity exercise. This does not mean to begin doing only high-intensity exercise because for optimal performance you need to do a mixture of high-intensity and low-intensity. The goal is to always keep your body guessing.

As for question two, unless you are a professional athlete or training for a highly competitive event in which you need to always maximize performance, the best time for you to workout is when you can be the most consistent. If that is in the morning, workout in the morning. If that is during lunch, then workout during lunch. As mentioned in Day 1, your commitment, consistency, and candor are requirements to achieving your health and fitness goals.

To eliminate all excuses that prevent cardio, here are ten body weight cardio exercises you can do at home, in the gym, in a hotel room, etc. Get your cardio in, no excuses. Have fun!

Day 13 - Cardio - Movement Towards your FinishLine

BODYWEIGHT CARDIO
Candice McField Fitness

| 2 sets per exercise | 60 seconds per set | 60 seconds rest between sets |

Equipment: Bodyweight

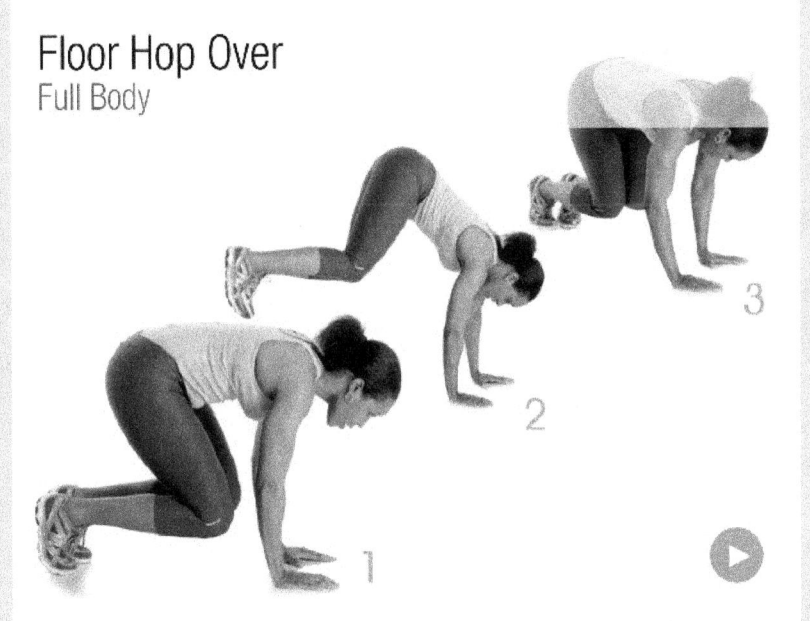

Floor Hop Over
Full Body

1. Start with your hands and toes on the floor, hips raised.
2. Hop both feet up and over to one side as you keep your hands on the floor.
- Repeat on the other side

scan the code to view a video of the workout

#	REPS	WEIGHT	TIME	NOTES
1			60.0	
2			60.0	

© 2020. Candice McField Fitness, LLC. All rights reserved. No part of this publication may be reproduced, distributed, or transmitted in any form, without prior written permission of Candice McField Fitness, LLC. User represents that he/she has consulted with a Physician regarding User's potential use of this workout, prior to beginning the workout, and that the physician consents to User's performance of the workout. The content of the workout and any information otherwise obtained by user through the workout is provided for information purposes only and User uses such information and content AT THE VOLUNTARY, SOLE RISK OF THE USER. USER RELEASES AND RELIEVES, AND AGREES TO RELEASE AND RELIEVE, CANDICE MCFIELD FITNESS, LLC. AND LAUNCHCRATE PUBLISHING, LLC. OF ANY AND ALL LIABILITY FOR ANY INJURIES, CLAIMS OR DAMAGES ARISING OUT OF USER'S USE OF THE SERVICE.

BODYWEIGHT CARDIO
Candice McField Fitness

| 2 sets per exercise | 60 seconds per set | 60 seconds rest between sets |

Equipment: Bodyweight

Ankle Over Knee
Full Body

- Stand with your feet together and your arms by your sides.
1. While jogging, raise your foot over your opposite knee.
2. Rapidly switch feet and raise your foot over your opposite knee as high as possible.

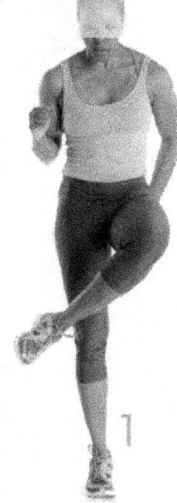

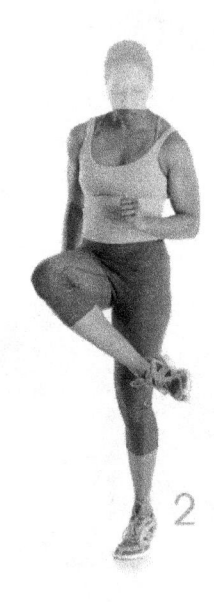

scan the code to view a video of the workout

#	REPS	WEIGHT	TIME	NOTES
1			60.0	
2			60.0	

© 2020. Candice McField Fitness, LLC. All rights reserved. No part of this publication may be reproduced, distributed, or transmitted in any form, without prior written permission of Candice McField Fitness, LLC. User represents that he/she has consulted with a Physician regarding User's potential use of this workout, prior to beginning the workout, and that the physician consents to User's performance of the workout. The content of the workout and any information otherwise obtained by user through the workout is provided for information purposes only and User uses such information and content AT THE VOLUNTARY, SOLE RISK OF THE USER. USER RELEASES AND RELIEVES, AND AGREES TO RELEASE AND RELIEVE, CANDICE MCFIELD FITNESS, LLC. AND LAUNCHCRATE PUBLISHING, LLC. OF ANY AND ALL LIABILITY FOR ANY INJURIES, CLAIMS OR DAMAGES ARISING OUT OF USER'S USE OF THE SERVICE.

Day 13 - Cardio - Movement Towards your Finish Line

BODYWEIGHT CARDIO
Candice McField Fitness

| 2 sets per exercise | 60 seconds per set | 60 seconds rest between sets |

Equipment: Bodyweight

Front Jumping Jacks
Full Body

scan the code to view a video of the workout

- Stand with your feet together and your arms by your sides.
1. Jump up, splitting your feet front to back while simultaneously swinging one arm forward and up to shoulder height, as the other arm lowers back and behind.
2. Reverse the direction of the movement.

#	REPS	WEIGHT	TIME	NOTES
1			60.0	
2			60.0	

© 2020. Candice McField Fitness, LLC. All rights reserved. No part of this publication may be reproduced, distributed, or transmitted in any form, without prior written permission of Candice McField Fitness, LLC. User represents that he/she has consulted with a Physician regarding User's potential use of this workout, prior to beginning the workout, and that the physician consents to User's performance of the workout. The content of the workout and any information otherwise obtained by user through the workout is provided for information purposes only and User uses such information and content AT THE VOLUNTARY, SOLE RISK OF THE USER. USER RELEASES AND RELIEVES, AND AGREES TO RELEASE AND RELIEVE, CANDICE MCFIELD FITNESS, LLC. AND LAUNCHCRATE PUBLISHING, LLC. OF ANY AND ALL LIABILITY FOR ANY INJURIES, CLAIMS OR DAMAGES ARISING OUT OF USER'S USE OF THE SERVICE.

BODYWEIGHT CARDIO
Candice McField Fitness

2 sets per exercise | **60 seconds** per set | **60 seconds** rest between sets

Equipment: Bodyweight

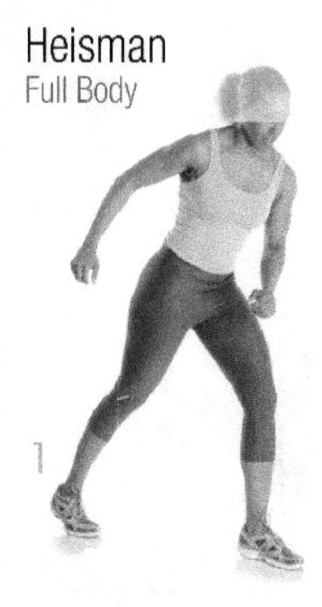

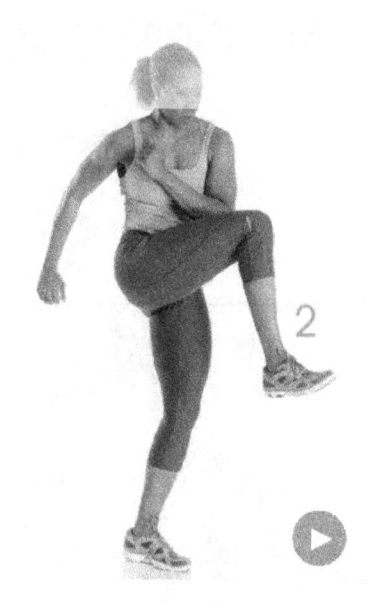

Heisman
Full Body

scan the code to view a video of the workout

- Stand with your arms by your sides.
1. Step back with one leg as you twist your torso to the opposite side.
2. Push off your front foot to bring the back leg forward, bending your knee and twisting your torso back to the other side.
- Complete all reps on one side before switching to the other side.

#	REPS	WEIGHT	TIME	NOTES
1			60.0	
2			60.0	

© 2020. Candice McField Fitness, LLC. All rights reserved. No part of this publication may be reproduced, distributed, or transmitted in any form, without prior written permission of Candice McField Fitness, LLC. User represents that he/she has consulted with a Physician regarding User's potential use of this workout, prior to beginning the workout, and that the physician consents to User's performance of the workout. The content of the workout and any information otherwise obtained by user through the workout is provided for information purposes only and User uses such information and content AT THE VOLUNTARY, SOLE RISK OF THE USER. USER RELEASES AND RELIEVES, AND AGREES TO RELEASE AND RELIEVE, CANDICE MCFIELD FITNESS, LLC. AND LAUNCHCRATE PUBLISHING, LLC. OF ANY AND ALL LIABILITY FOR ANY INJURIES, CLAIMS OR DAMAGES ARISING OUT OF USER'S USE OF THE SERVICE.

Day 13 - Cardio - Movement Towards your FinishLine

BODYWEIGHT CARDIO
Candice McField Fitness

2 sets per exercise
60 seconds per set
60 seconds rest between sets

Equipment: Bodyweight

Two Way Jump
Full Body

1. Stand with your feet together, arms by your sides.
2. Jump your feet out to the sides, about 3 feet.
3. Jump your feet back in together in the middle.
4. Jump to split your feet front to back.
- Jump back to the start position and repeat.

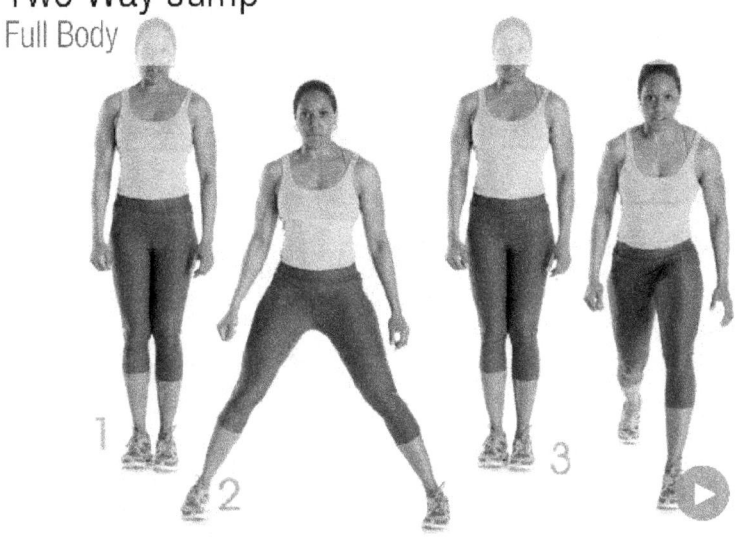

scan the code to view a video of the workout

#	REPS	WEIGHT	TIME	NOTES
1			60.0	
2			60.0	

© 2020. Candice McField Fitness, LLC. All rights reserved. No part of this publication may be reproduced, distributed, or transmitted in any form, without prior written permission of Candice McField Fitness, LLC. User represents that he/she has consulted with a Physician regarding User's potential use of this workout, prior to beginning the workout, and that the physician consents to User's performance of the workout. The content of the workout and any information otherwise obtained by user through the workout is provided for information purposes only and User uses such information and content AT THE VOLUNTARY, SOLE RISK OF THE USER. USER RELEASES AND RELIEVES, AND AGREES TO RELEASE AND RELIEVE, CANDICE MCFIELD FITNESS, LLC. AND LAUNCHCRATE PUBLISHING, LLC. OF ANY AND ALL LIABILITY FOR ANY INJURIES, CLAIMS OR DAMAGES ARISING OUT OF USER'S USE OF THE SERVICE.

BODYWEIGHT CARDIO
Candice McField Fitness

2 sets per exercise | **60 seconds** per set | **60 seconds** rest between sets

Equipment: Bodyweight

Lateral Jump Taps
Full Body

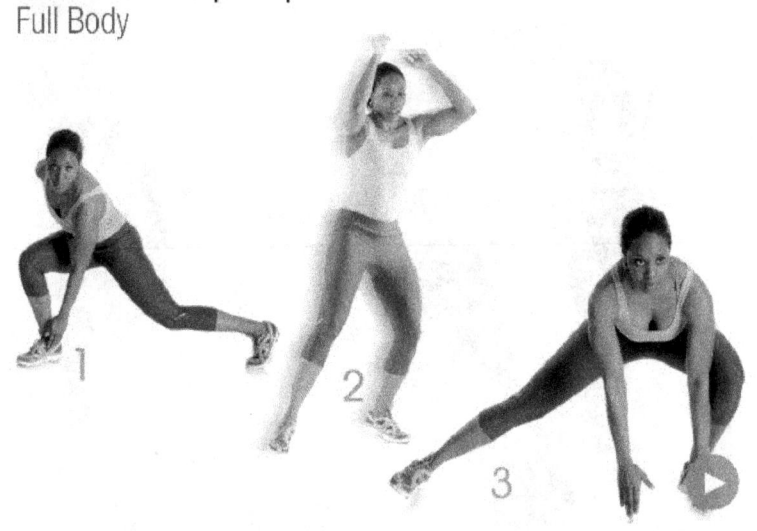

scan the code to view a video of the workout

- Stand with your arms by your sides.
1. Tap the floor on the side of one foot with your opposite hand. Jump laterally to the other side as you raise both arms overhead.
2. Land in a partial squat, tap your other hand down towards the outside foot. Quickly jump back to the original side, raising both arms overhead
- Continue jumping back and forth from side to side, tapping your hand to the opposite foot each time.

#	REPS	WEIGHT	TIME	NOTES
1			60.0	
2			60.0	

© 2020. Candice McField Fitness, LLC. All rights reserved. No part of this publication may be reproduced, distributed, or transmitted in any form, without prior written permission of Candice McField Fitness, LLC. User represents that he/she has consulted with a Physician regarding User's potential use of this workout, prior to beginning the workout, and that the physician consents to User's performance of the workout. The content of the workout and any information otherwise obtained by user through the workout is provided for information purposes only and User uses such information and content AT THE VOLUNTARY, SOLE RISK OF THE USER. USER RELEASES AND RELIEVES, AND AGREES TO RELEASE AND RELIEVE, CANDICE MCFIELD FITNESS, LLC. AND LAUNCHCRATE PUBLISHING, LLC. OF ANY AND ALL LIABILITY FOR ANY INJURIES, CLAIMS OR DAMAGES ARISING OUT OF USER'S USE OF THE SERVICE.

Day 13 - Cardio - Movement Towards your Finish Line

BODYWEIGHT CARDIO
Candice McField Fitness

2 sets per exercise | **60 seconds** per set | **60 seconds** rest between sets

Equipment: Bodyweight

Quick Feet
Full Body

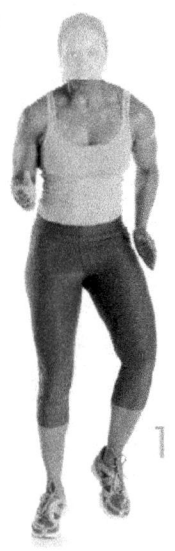

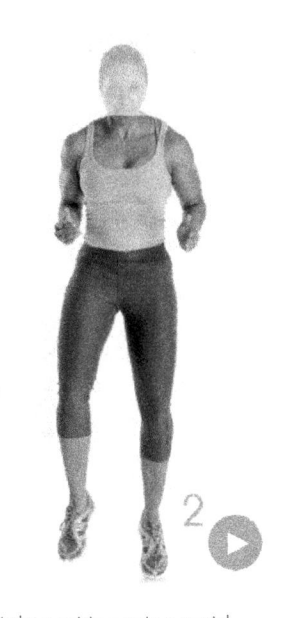

scan the code to view a video of the workout

1. Run on the spot in an upright position using rapid short steps, holding your hands up at chest level.

#	REPS	WEIGHT	TIME	NOTES
1			60.0	
2			60.0	

© 2020. Candice McField Fitness, LLC. All rights reserved. No part of this publication may be reproduced, distributed, or transmitted in any form, without prior written permission of Candice McField Fitness, LLC. User represents that he/she has consulted with a Physician regarding User's potential use of this workout, prior to beginning the workout, and that the physician consents to User's performance of the workout. The content of the workout and any information otherwise obtained by user through the workout is provided for information purposes only and User uses such information and content AT THE VOLUNTARY, SOLE RISK OF THE USER. USER RELEASES AND RELIEVES, AND AGREES TO RELEASE AND RELIEVE, CANDICE MCFIELD FITNESS, LLC. AND LAUNCHCRATE PUBLISHING, LLC. OF ANY AND ALL LIABILITY FOR ANY INJURIES, CLAIMS OR DAMAGES ARISING OUT OF USER'S USE OF THE SERVICE.

BODYWEIGHT CARDIO
Candice McField Fitness

| 2 sets per exercise | 60 seconds per set | 60 seconds rest between sets |

Equipment: Bodyweight

Speed Skater
Full Body

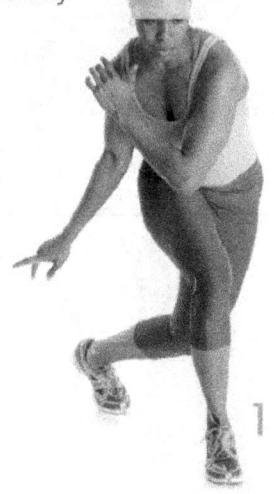

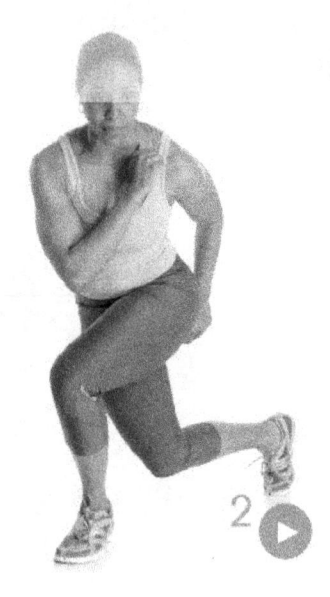

scan the code to view a video of the workout

1. Stand with one leg extended out behind and across the other leg, arms reaching to the same side.
2. Push off your front leg, jumping to the other side. As you land, switch your legs and immediately jump back.
- Swing your arms as if you are skating.

#	REPS	WEIGHT	TIME	NOTES
1			60.0	
2			60.0	

© 2020. Candice McField Fitness, LLC. All rights reserved. No part of this publication may be reproduced, distributed, or transmitted in any form, without prior written permission of Candice McField Fitness, LLC. User represents that he/she has consulted with a Physician regarding User's potential use of this workout, prior to beginning the workout, and that the physician consents to User's performance of the workout. The content of the workout and any information otherwise obtained by user through the workout is provided for information purposes only and User uses such information and content AT THE VOLUNTARY, SOLE RISK OF THE USER. USER RELEASES AND RELIEVES, AND AGREES TO RELEASE AND RELIEVE, CANDICE MCFIELD FITNESS, LLC. AND LAUNCHCRATE PUBLISHING, LLC. OF ANY AND ALL LIABILITY FOR ANY INJURIES, CLAIMS OR DAMAGES ARISING OUT OF USER'S USE OF THE SERVICE.

Day 13 - Cardio - Movement Towards your FinishLine

BODYWEIGHT CARDIO
Candice McField Fitness

| 2 sets per exercise | 60 seconds per set | 60 seconds rest between sets |

Equipment: Bodyweight

Outside Hand to Ankle
Full Body

- Stand with your feet together and with your arms by your sides.
1. While jogging, laterally raise your foot as high as possible, tapping the outside of your ankle.
2. Rapidly switch feet, then repeat on the opposite side.
- Continue jogging forward, repeating the movement.

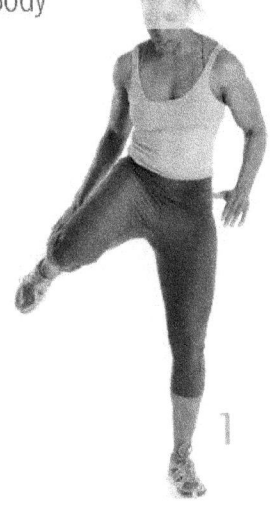

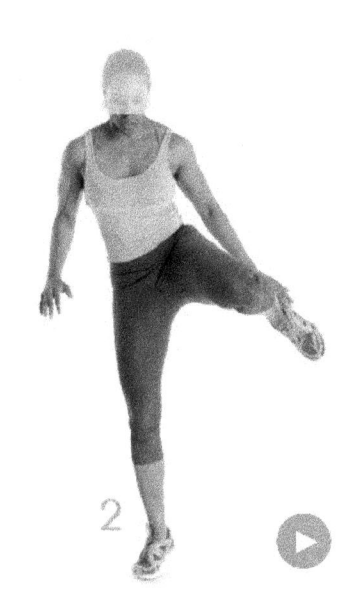

scan the code to view a video of the workout

#	REPS	WEIGHT	TIME	NOTES
1			60.0	
2			60.0	

© 2020. Candice McField Fitness, LLC. All rights reserved. No part of this publication may be reproduced, distributed, or transmitted in any form, without prior written permission of Candice McField Fitness, LLC. User represents that he/she has consulted with a Physician regarding User's potential use of this workout, prior to beginning the workout, and that the physician consents to User's performance of the workout. The content of the workout and any information otherwise obtained by user through the workout is provided for information purposes only and User uses such information and content AT THE VOLUNTARY, SOLE RISK OF THE USER. USER RELEASES AND RELIEVES, AND AGREES TO RELEASE AND RELIEVE, CANDICE MCFIELD FITNESS, LLC. AND LAUNCHCRATE PUBLISHING, LLC. OF ANY AND ALL LIABILITY FOR ANY INJURIES, CLAIMS OR DAMAGES ARISING OUT OF USER'S USE OF THE SERVICE.

BODYWEIGHT CARDIO
Candice McField Fitness

2 sets per exercise | **60 seconds** per set | **60 seconds** rest between sets

Equipment: Bodyweight

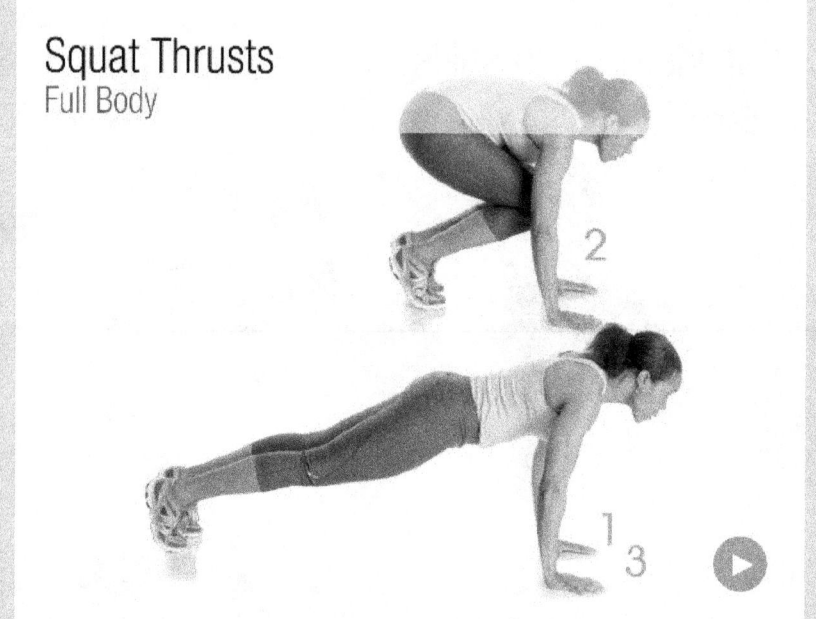

Squat Thrusts
Full Body

1. Start in the top position of a push up with your legs and arms straight.
2. Jump your feet in, bringing your knees to your chest as you keep your hands on the floor.
3. Jump your feet back out to a straight position and repeat.

scan the code to view a video of the workout

#	REPS	WEIGHT	TIME	NOTES
1			60.0	
2			60.0	

© 2020. Candice McField Fitness, LLC. All rights reserved. No part of this publication may be reproduced, distributed, or transmitted in any form, without prior written permission of Candice McField Fitness, LLC. User represents that he/she has consulted with a Physician regarding User's potential use of this workout, prior to beginning the workout, and that the physician consents to User's performance of the workout. The content of the workout and any information otherwise obtained by user through the workout is provided for information purposes only and User uses such information and content AT THE VOLUNTARY, SOLE RISK OF THE USER. USER RELEASES AND RELIEVES, AND AGREES TO RELEASE AND RELIEVE, CANDICE MCFIELD FITNESS, LLC. AND LAUNCHCRATE PUBLISHING, LLC. OF ANY AND ALL LIABILITY FOR ANY INJURIES, CLAIMS OR DAMAGES ARISING OUT OF USER'S USE OF THE SERVICE.

Day 13 - Cardio - Movement Towards your Finish Line

Day 13
Unlocking My Optimal Performance

Moment of Truth: You cannot build and maintain an incredible physique without doing both cardio and strength training.

Quote to Remember: "Think of your workouts as important meetings that you've scheduled with yourself. Bosses don't cancel."

— Anonymous

Challenge to Implement: Identify two health benefits of cardio you would like to improve. Then identify two ways you really enjoy doing cardio. Commit to executing those two ways at least three times per week for 30 minutes each day.

Soli Deo Gloria and *Arise!*®

Candice

Two health benefits of cardio I would like to improve:

1)

2)

Two ways I enjoy doing cardio are:

1)

2)

Day 14

Sleep Essentials

My home church is unconventional. We sometimes break into small discussion groups after the sermon to pray together and discuss applicable questions related to the sermon. One Sunday, a member mentioned a great practical tip she does before she begins her prayer/meditation time. She takes five minutes of stillness and quietness before she goes into prayer. I remember thinking how cool of an idea that was. Instead of immediately going into prayer, take five minutes, clear all your thoughts, and really listen for what God is telling you. Oftentimes, our eagerness to jump into the list of demands, requests, and worries we have for God makes us forget to listen for His voice and have Him talk to us. I immediately put this five minute rule into practice. The clarity that comes when you slow down, stop, and listen to hear what God is telling you truly is amazing.

Another incredible way to hear God's voice is through biblical fasting. Fasting is abstinence from food or something else for a period, to focus your thoughts and worship on God. When faced with big decisions, I often fast and look for confirmation. I fast using Psalms 28:6-7 as my key verse and I look for confirmation in three ways: through His word, through spiritual counselors, and, through circumstances. Regardless of the decision or outcome, I find comfort in

Psalms 28:6 7.

*Praise the Lord!
For he has heard my cry for mercy.
The Lord is my strength and shield.
I trust him with all my heart.
He helps me, and my heart is filled with joy.
I burst out in songs of thanksgiving.*

Day 14
Unlocking My Optimal Performance

Moment of Truth: Take time each day to be still and to honor God.

Verse to Remember: *"Be still, and know that I am God!"*
Psalms 46:10 (NLT)

Challenge to Implement: *Before you begin your prayer and meditation time, begin taking five minutes to listen to what God wants to tell you! If you are already doing this then add an additional 5 minutes to your time.*

Soli Deo Gloria and *Arise!*®

Candice

During my first few years as a figure competitor, I would purposely live on 4 hours of sleep. I vividly remember telling my trainer, "I do not need the traditional 7-8 hours." He used to get on me and stay on me about this because he knew what I failed to realize at the time. Sleep is critical to achieving optimal performance in everything you do

Day 14 - Sleep Essentials

in life and research proves this. It was not until I attended a meeting where the keynote speaker was a renowned sleep doctor. He emphasized, how for anyone who wants to be successful, sleep is a necessity, not a luxury. The potential for peak performance is a given every morning, with adequate sleep.

Everyone should know exactly how much sleep he or she requires to feel wide awake, dynamic, and energetic all day. Everyone should know the strategies and techniques for getting quality sleep for maximum daytime performance as well as how to cope with sleep deprivation when it does occur.

If you are getting less than eight hours of sleep per night, fall asleep instantly, or need an alarm clock to wake up, you are chronically sleep-deprived – and possibly ignorant to how sleepy and ineffective you are, or how dynamic you *could* be with adequate sleep. Millions of people are in this same position. At least 50% of the American adult population suffers from sleep deprivation.

Most of us need at least one more hour of sleep than we get each night. While the consequences of gradual, continuous sleep deprivation might not be immediately apparent, over time, exhaustion takes its toll on mood, performance, and health. Eventually, it affects every aspect of your life.

How do you become less sleep deprived? Follow our Essentials of Sleep Principles and Great Sleep Strategies.

Essentials of Sleep Principles

1. **Establish a regular sleep schedule.**
   Be consistent with your bedtime and waking time, even on weekends.

2. **Get an adequate amount of sleep every night.**
   Strive to get 7-8 hours of sleep each night. For most people, this means getting at least sixty to ninety minutes more sleep than you are presently getting.

3. **Get continuous sleep.**
   To maximize rejuvenation, try to sleep in one continuous block versus multiple short blocks of time. For instance, you will feel more rejuvenated if you sleep 7-8 hours straight, versus sleeping a few hours at a time.

4. **Make up for lost sleep.**
   Executing these first three essentials are doable but I also recognize how difficult it will be for some of you to do them consistently. Therefore, make up for any lost sleep as soon as possible. In addition, return to your regular sleep schedule as soon as possible.

Great Sleep Strategies

Learn to value sleep	Take a warm bath before bed
Exercise to stay fit	Establish a bedtime ritual
Eat clean	Have pleasurable sexual activity
Reduce stress as much as possible	Maintain a relaxing atmosphere in the bedroom
Keep mentally stimulated during the day	Clear your mind at bedtime
Reduce caffeine intake	Try some bedtime relaxation techniques
Avoid alcohol near bedtime	Avoid trying too hard to get to sleep

Day 14 - Sleep Essentials

Two of the top ways to get better sleep is to exercise and to eat clean. Research studies show exercise is directly correlated to better sleep. Exercise reduces stress, anxiety, and insomnia while raising endorphin levels. Endorphins are mood enhancers that reduce pain, relax muscles, suppress appetite, and produce feelings of general well-being. People who exercise experience deeper, more restful sleep. Furthermore, exercise elevates your core body temperature. An ensuing drop in body temperature at bedtime, five or six hours after a vigorous workout, induces drowsiness and deeper sleep. It is worth nothing that exercise releases adrenaline. Therefore, you may not want to work out within three hours of bedtime. Doing so may cause high alertness, making it difficult for your body to relax enough to induce sleep.

In general, healthy people sleep better and being healthy involves eating clean. On Days 5 and 6, I stressed the importance of eating small, clean meals throughout the day. I also listed sample daily meals and explained eating clean. As you implement the strategies shared on Days 5 and 6, avoid eating large or heavy meals within four or five hours of going to bed. While a substantial intake of food can make you feel drowsy initially, you may toss and turn during the night. You are also likely to gain weight by eating too late in the day to burn off the calories. When you eat a big meal, the body dumps a large amount of insulin into your system, which helps store fat. If you add that to the inactivity of sleep, the body will store much more fat than usual. Therefore, it is more important to be mindful of what you eat late at night rather than what time you eat at night. If you are hungry late at night eat lean protein and vegetables.

Lastly, avoid foods that cause indigestion, gas, or heartburn. Consuming these foods will almost ensure a restless night. Some examples of foods to avoid include pickles, garlic, fatty, and spicy foods.

As For Me and My Body

Day 14
Unlocking My Optimal Performance

Moment of Truth: Sleep is critical to achieve optimal performance with everything you do in life!

Quote to Remember: *"Sleep is the golden chain that ties health and our bodies together."*
— Thomas Dekker

Challenge to Implement: Identify and focus on improving one of the Essentials of Sleep Principles. Set an act ion plan to achieve that goal. Next, list two great sleep strategies you will use to get better sleep.

Soli Deo Gloria and *Arise!*®

Candice

The essential rule I will focus on to improve my sleep is:

One action I can take to achieve this goal is:

Two great sleep strategies I will use to get better sleep:

1)

2)

Week 3

Day 15

Breakfast Sets the Standard

One of the best gifts I ever received was a Bible from my dad when I graduated high school. Inside, he wrote a message to me that is beyond special, one that I will someday pass on to my kids. He wrote:

"To my daughter Candice,
Keep Jesus as the center of your life and let his light shine in you for all to see.

Remember to give God and the Lord Jesus Christ the praise for all of your accomplishments.

When you experience trials and tribulations remember God has not forsaken you. Be Patient and He will see you through.

Proverbs 3:5-6
Trust in the Lord with all your heart.
And lean not on your own understanding.
In all your ways acknowledge Him, and He shall direct your paths.

Read all of Proverbs Chapter 3 to know God's principles and guidance for you.

As For Me and My Body

When you do not know what to pray you can always pray the Lord's prayer Matthew 6:19-13.

Sharing God's goodness and His holy Word and my love as your father." Quinton T. McField 5/25/99

What a stunning and incredibly powerful message from the man dearest to my heart. I did not understand the significance of this gift when I received it, but later in life it made perfect sense. This gift never loses its unsurpassed giving power. Just as trusting in the Lord with all your heart sets the foundation for your walk with Christ, eating breakfast everyday sets the standard for making clean eating a lifestyle.

Day 15
Unlocking My Optimal Performance

Moment of Truth: Trusting in the Lord with all your heart is the foundation of your walk with Christ.

Verse to Remember: *"Trust in the Lord with all your heart. And lean not on your own understanding."*

Proverbs 3:5 (NLT)

Challenge to Implement: *Trust in the Lord with all your heart. Let go of all control over one more area in your life and give it to Him. If you have successfully executed Day 11's challenge, then add one more area to give to God. If you have not executed Day 11's challenge yet, make it your focus today.*

Soli Deo Gloria and *Arise!*®

Candice

Day 15 - Breakfast Sets the Standard

Breakfast is the most important meal of the day. It sets the tone and standard for eating habits, productivity, and energy levels for the rest of the day.

I have a confession. Breakfast is by far my favorite meal of the day and I eat it religiously every morning. Earlier this week, an anomaly occurred. I felt extremely lazy and warmed up leftovers from dining out rather than making my standard breakfast. My microwaved breakfast was not the healthiest.

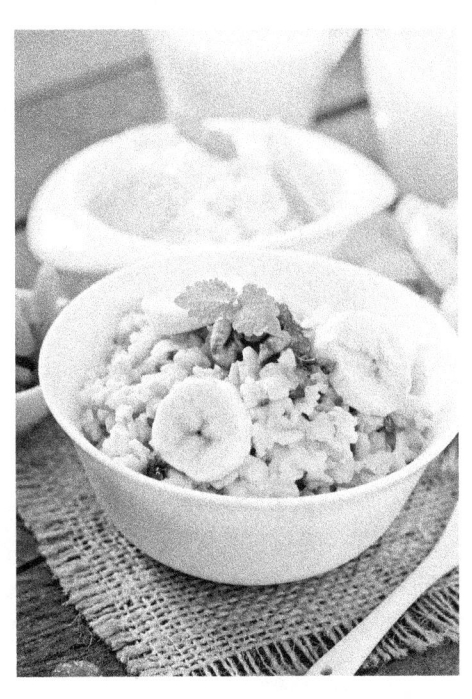

It was orange chicken and fried rice as compared to my standard 2 eggs, 2 egg whites with hot cereal. My unhealthy choice first thing in the morning triggered me to make poor choices for two other meals that same day. Eating a healthier breakfast often influences how you eat for the rest of the day. Although it may be rare, I too, fall off the bandwagon at times. More importantly, I get back on as soon as I can.

Falling off the bandwagon is the most common pitfall I hear from people. They will tell me, "Candice, I had donuts for breakfast, so I cheated the rest of the day." We are our own toughest critics and tend to beat ourselves up for one slip up or failure. Remember, there is no perfection requirement. If you have a "bad" meal, simply count it as one of your cheat meals for the week instead of blowing the entire day. I cannot stress to you enough how important it is to get back on the bandwagon for your next meal. Do not wait an entire day.

Waiting a day later often turns into a week later. You may say, "On Monday, I will start back up." Unfortunately, Monday comes, then it goes. This frame of thinking becomes a cycle of "next Mondays." Trust me avoid this perpetual downward spiral and get back on the bandwagon after one cheat meal. Although breakfast is only one of your five to six daily meals, it should provide approximately 25% of your nutritional requirements each day. A practical guide you can follow is to consume a complex carbohydrate, a lean protein, plus a fruit and/or vegetable each morning.

One of the best complex carb options in the morning is to eat a hot cereal, such as oatmeal. The digestive system breaks down hot cereal very slowly which means you will feel fuller, longer. The protein helps stimulate your metabolism, improves muscle mass and recovery, and reduces body fat. The fruit and vegetable will provide an alkaline load to the blood. Since both proteins and complex carbohydrates present acid loads to the blood, it is important to balance these acids with alkaline rich vegetables and fruits. Too much acid and not enough alkalinity means the loss of bone strength and muscle mass.

Following is a list of protein, complex carbohydrate, fruit and vegetable options. The list is not exhaustive. Instead, I provided it to offer ideas of what to create for breakfast and to help you understand what category various foods fall under.

Day 13 – Breakfast Sets the Standard

	Proteins	Veggies	Fruits	Carbs	Fats
Lean Meats	Beef tenderloin Bison Chicken breast Ground turkey Pork Tenderloin Turkey Venison	Artichoke Asparagus Bok choy Broccoli Brussels sprouts Cabbage Carrots	Apples Avocados Berries Citrus fruits Dried fruits (in moderation) Grapefruit Grapes	Amaranth Barley Beans (kidney, navy, pinto, soy) Brown rice Buckwheat Cereals Chickpeas	Animal Fats (eaten in eggs) Almonds Avocados Cashews Coconut Oil Cold-water fish Fish Oil
Fish	Canned Salmon, packed in water Canned Tuna, packed in water Cod Halibut Roughy Salmon Tilapia	Cauliflower Celery Cucumbers Eggplant Kale Lettuce Okra	Kiwi Lychee Mango Melons Oranges Papaya	Couscous (wheat or rice) Lentils Multi-grain Millet Mixed beans Oatmeal Oats	Flax Seeds/Oil Hazelnut Oil Nut and nut butters Nuts and nut butters Olive Oil Palm Oil Pecans
Eggs	Egg whites Occasional whole eggs	Onions Spinach	Passion fruit Pears	Potatoes Quinoa	Pumpkinseed Oil Safflower Oil
Low Fat Dairy	Low-fat Cottage cheese Fat-free, plain yogurt Parmesan cheese String cheese	Tomatoes Turnip greens Watermelon Zucchini	Plums Pomegranate	Realistic Spinaches Sweet potatoes Wheat germ Wheat or processed grains Whole grain bread Whole grain or rice pasta Whole grains in appropriate size Yams	Vegetable Oils Walnuts
Vegetarian	Tofu Hemp of all kinds Chickpeas Kale Lentils Seitan Soy bean Soy Burgers Soy Jerky Soy Sausage Tempeh				
Protein Supplements	Casein Milk protein isolate Whey				
Other	Natural nut butters (almond, cocoa, peanut) Nut-milks (rice, soy, oat, almond, cashew or any milk) Unsalted nuts of all kinds				

Candice McField
Animal
UNIVERSITY
UNLOCK OPTIMAL PERFORMANCE

As For Me and My Body

Day 15
Unlocking My Optimal Performance

Moment of Truth: Breakfast sets the tone and standard for your eating habits, productivity, and energy levels for the rest of the day.

Quote to Remember: *"Breakfast is everything. The beginning, the first thing. It is the mouthful that is the commitment to a new day, a continuing life."*

— A.A. Gill

Challenge to Implement: *Commit to eating breakfast five out of seven days to start. If you are eating breakfast daily, commit to eating a healthier breakfast.*

Soli Deo Gloria and *Arise!*®

Candice

I currently do not eat breakfast:

I commit to eating breakfast at least 5 out of 7 days per week starting on _____.

Once I begin eating breakfast 5 days per week, I will increase my commitment to 7 days.

I currently eat breakfast 7 days a week:

Identify 2 ways you can make your breakfast healthier

1)

2)

Day 16

Quenching Thirst

The Pursuit of God by A.W. Tozer is one of the best spiritual books that I have read. I highly recommend it as a must read for many reasons. In the first chapter, Tozer begins:

> "We pursue God because, and only because, He has first put an urge within us that spurs us to the pursuit. "No man can come to me," said our Lord, "except the Father which hath sent me draw him," and it is by this very prevenient drawing that God takes from us every vestige of credit for the act of coming. The impulse to pursue God originates with God, but the outworking of that impulse is our following hard after Him; and all the time we are pursuing Him we are already in His hand: "Thy right hand upholdeth me."
>
> The whole transaction of religious conversion has been made mechanical and spiritless...Christ may be "received" without creating any special love for Him in the soul of the receiver. The man is "saved," but he is not hungry nor thirsty after God. In fact, he is specifically taught to be satisfied and encouraged to be content with little.
>
> The modern scientist has lost God amid the wonders of His world; we Christians are in real danger of losing God

amid the wonders of His Word. We have almost forgotten that God is a Person and, as such, can be cultivated as any person can. It is inherent in personality to be able to know other personalities, but full knowledge of one personality by another cannot be achieved in one encounter. It is only after long and loving mental intercourse that the full possibilities of both can be explored."

We cultivate all other relationships, why not do the same with Christ? Just as water is essential for the body, we must thirst for Christ. My favorite Christian rapper is Dillon Chase. One of my favorite songs by him is called, *The Pursuit*. Here is part of the chorus.

> *"I'll pursue Him 'til my lungs collapse*
> *and if I don't it's probably because the Son came back*
> *I can't stop (can't stop)*
> *I won't stop (won't stop)*
> *I've been called (been called)*
> *but I got to pursue Him (heeey)*
> *You follow God with all you got say let's go*
> *Let's follow God with all we got say let's go."*

Let our thirst for God spark us to follow hard after Him until our lungs collapse or until He comes back.

Day 16

Unlocking My Optimal Performance

Moment of Truth: We cultivate our relationships; we must do the same with our relationship with Christ!

Verse to Remember: *"As the deer longs for streams of water, so I long for you, O God. I thirst for God, the living God. When can I go and stand before him?"*

Psalms 42:1-2 (NLT)

Challenge to Implement: *Cultivate, your relationship with God by writing Him a love letter. Also, I encourage you to read the book The Pursuit of God by A.W. Tozer.*

Soli Deo Gloria and *Arise!*®

Candice

Water is as important as oxygen, and dehydration is powerful. Adults can survive without food for weeks but can only survive for up to 10 days without water. Water makes up 50 70% of our total body weight and is the main facilitator of digestion. Therefore, consuming 3 liters of water daily is ideal.

Functions of Water	
Main facilitator of digestion	Nutrient Absorption
Protecting Vital Organs	Regulating Body Temperature
Medium for All Biochemical Reactions	Maintaining High Blood Volume for Optimal Performance

PERCENTAGE OF BODY WATER LOST

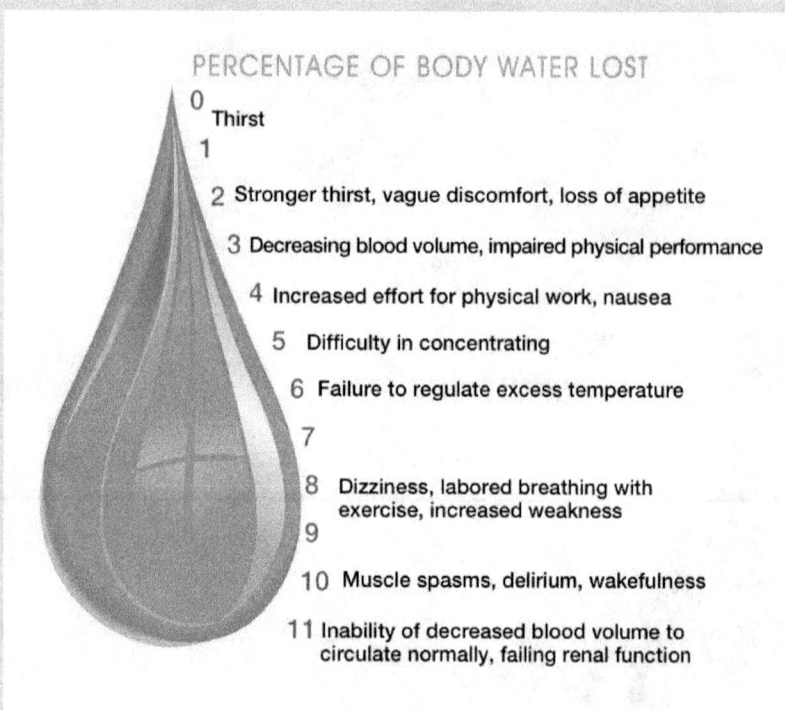

- 0 Thirst
- 1
- 2 Stronger thirst, vague discomfort, loss of appetite
- 3 Decreasing blood volume, impaired physical performance
- 4 Increased effort for physical work, nausea
- 5 Difficulty in concentrating
- 6 Failure to regulate excess temperature
- 7
- 8 Dizziness, labored breathing with exercise, increased weakness
- 9
- 10 Muscle spasms, delirium, wakefulness
- 11 Inability of decreased blood volume to circulate normally, failing renal function

Thirst is a poor indicator of hydration because it goes undetected until we have lost 1-2% of our body's water. Decreasing your total body water by just 1% can decrease your overall effectiveness by as much as 10%. Loss of only 10% causes severe disorders while loss of 20% can cause death. If you are thirsty, you are already dehydrated.

Ways We Dehydrate	
Breathing	Consuming toxins
Stress	Diarrhea
Digestion	Vomiting
Sweating	Fever
Pregnancy	Chronic illness
Aging	Sun exposure

Day 16 - Quenching Thirst

Growing	Exercise
Obesity	Not drinking enough water
Diets high in processed foods	Decreased mineral water
Medications	Burns

There are many drinks on grocery shelves believed to be great hydrating sources. Beware of the following:

Drinks that will Dehydrate You	
Caffeine	Soda
Fruit juices	Tea
Soft drinks	Coffee
Energy drinks	Alcohol

In addition, utilize sport drinks and artificially flavored water sparingly. Sports drinks are abnormally high in sugar, making the high sugar and carbohydrate consumption, often not worth the calories. Although touted to be beneficial for hydration, studies have found **the additives in sports drinks have no effect on water absorption in our bodies**. Nothing gets more water into your system than water. However, a good place and time to utilize sports drinks are when you are exercising for extended periods, like running a marathon.

Artificially flavored water is another popular item. It is important that you read the label because many contain artificial flavors, colors, sugars, and salts -- all of which you want to steer clear. The excuse I hear most for why people do not drink water is that it has no flavor. It is time to drop the excuses and begin adding natural pizzazz to your water using fruits and herbs.

Things to Add to your Water for Pizzazz	
Lemon slices	Lime slices
Cucumber slices	Orange slices
Strawberries	Unsweetened fruit juice
Caffeine-free herbal tea bags	Peppermint leaves

Day 16
Unlocking My Optimal Performance

Moment of Truth: Thirst is a poor indicator of hydration status because thirst usually is not perceived until 1-2% of body water is lost.

Quote to Remember: "Drinking water is as important as breathing oxygen."

— Collier Lunn

Challenge to Implement: Identify how much water you drink on a daily basis. The goal is to drink at least 3 liters per day. Identify something you drink that is actually dehydrating you. Identify one way to add pizzazz to your water.

Soli Deo Gloria and *Arise!*®

Candice

Quenching Thirst	
I drink _____ liters of water per day.	When I drink _____ it is really dehydrating me.
I can add pizzazz to my water by adding:	

Day 17

Range of Motion

The range of love God has for us is too big for us to understand fully. The breadth, depth, height, power, and presence of God's love exceeds our greatest imagination. In Ephesians 3:14-20, Paul beautifully exposits God's love for us in his prayer for our spiritual growth. He exclaims:

> "When I think of all this, I fall to my knees and pray to the Father, the Creator of everything in heaven and on earth. I pray that from his glorious, unlimited resources he will empower you with inner strength through his Spirit. Then Christ will make his home in your hearts as you trust in him. Your **roots** will grow down into God's love and keep you strong. And may you have the power to understand, as all God's people should, **how wide, how long, how high, and how deep his love is**. May you experience the love of Christ, though it is too great to understand fully. Then you will be made complete with all the fullness of life and power that comes from God. Now all glory to God, who is able, through his mighty power at work within us, to accomplish infinitely more than we might ask or think."

There was a plaque that read, "If you are going to pray, why worry? If you are going to worry, why pray," on my grandmother's room door. Before I became a believer, there was always something very special about those words on Granny's door. It was if I knew and believed it as truth before I was rooted in a real fellowship with Christ. It is amazing how life's puzzle pieces always come together, even if it is later in life. I made a note in my Bible regarding Verse 17, *"Your roots will grow down into God's love and keep you strong."* My note simply states, "Roots are planted in soil; our soil is Christ." When will we understand that because of who God is, the range of His love has no limits? God's love through Christ is immeasurable. The quote on Granny's door makes complete sense.

Just as God's range of love is immeasurable, having full range of motion in your muscles and joints is critical to unlocking your optimal performance.

Day 17
Unlocking My Optimal Performance

Moment of Truth: The range of love God has for us is too big for us to understand fully!

Verse to Remember: *"And may you have the power to understand, as all God's people should, how wide, how long, how high, and how deep his love is."*
Ephesians 3:18 (NLT)

Challenge to Implement: *Reflect on how wide, how long, how high, and how deep God's love has been for you. Pray a prayer of thanksgiving for His love.*

Soli Deo Gloria and *Arise!*®

Candice

Day 17 - Range of Motion

Flexibility is often the most neglected component of physical fitness. It is the ability to move joints through their normal full range of motion. An adequate degree of flexibility is important to prevent musculo-skeletal injuries and to maintain correct body posture. Flexibility helps balance muscle groups that might be overused during physical training sessions or because of poor posture. Factors affecting flexibility include age, gender, joint structure, muscle tendon attachments, muscle cross sectional area, body temperature, and pregnancy.

After age 25, flexibility tends to level off and thereafter begins to decline. However, significant improvements in flexibility can be achieved by following a sound training and flexibility program. Increasing and maintaining flexibility is an appropriate goal for all ages.

Reported Health Benefits of Flexibility

Increased physical efficiency	Improved muscular balance
Increased physical performance	Improved posture awareness
Increased blood supply to joints	Decreased risk of lower back pain
Improved nutrient exchange	Reduced muscular tension
Increased neuromuscular coordination	Enhanced exercise enjoyment

Despite working on your flexibility through daily stretching, inevitably, you will have some knots in your muscles that stretching alone cannot eliminate. For less than $20, there are two portable and incredible solutions: utilizing a foam roller and a tennis ball. Using these two items along with stretching daily, will greatly enhance your flexibility and reduce muscle soreness.

Foam rolling, also called myofascial release, is designed

to work out the knots in your muscles. Think of it as a self massage! The industry term for the knots in your muscles is called trigger points or myofascial adhesions. Myofascial adhesions can develop through stress, training, overuse, underuse, movement imbalances and injuries. They are essentially, points of constant tension and studies show addressing them can have a positive effect on your workouts, flexibility and reduce soreness. Ignoring them can lead to further dysfunction and may perpetuate and or cause injury. Depending on the foam intensity of your roller, utilizing a tennis ball is great for deeper trigger points and can be easily packed in any suitcase when you travel. Regardless if you are using a foam roller or tennis ball, find a sore spot and maintain pressure on it until it releases. Typically, this is 5-10 seconds. Then move the roller or tennis ball to another spot. When all your sore spots on the right side have been released, move over to your left side and repeat the process.

Benefits of Foam Rolling

Increased blood flow	Better range of motion
Restoring muscle length balance across joints	Relieving pain, soreness, and stiffness
Increased circulation and blood flow for faster recovery	Breaking up scar tissue and contusions
Increased flexibility which leads to lengthened muscles and a higher power threshold	

Each night for 10 to 15 minutes before bed, I stretch, use the foam roller, and then I use a tennis ball to work out any knots the foam roller did not eliminate. This routine has truly helped me to stay limber and has significantly helped an ongoing shoulder imbalance that I have.
Here is a stretching and foam roller routine that you can use daily. Stay flexible, knot free, and enjoy!

Day 17 - Range of Motion

Foam Roller
Candice McField Fitness

| 1 set per exercise | 30 seconds per set | 60 seconds rest between sets |

Equipment: Foam Roller

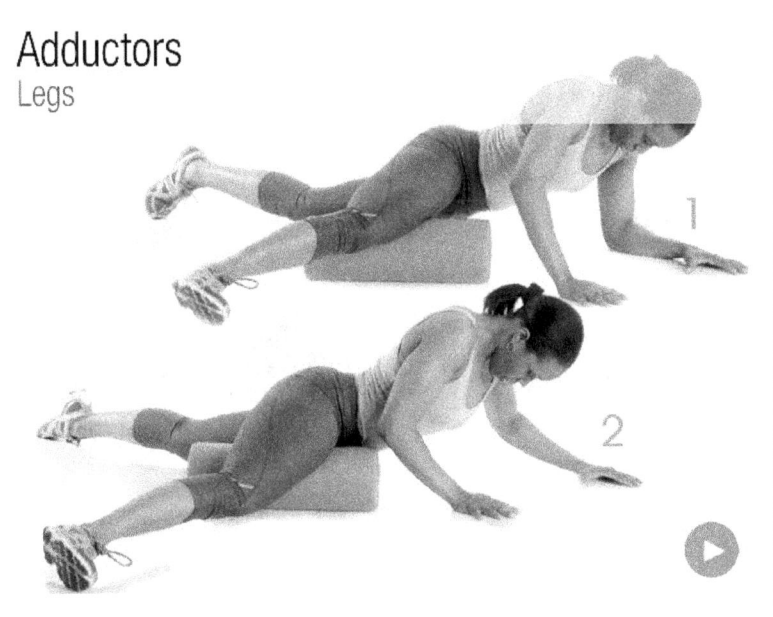

Adductors
Legs

1. Lie face down with a roller under your inner thigh and one leg bent at 90-degrees.
2. From your inside hip to your knee, roll back and forth along your inner thigh.
- Complete all reps on one side before switching to the other side.

scan the code to view a video of the workout

#	REPS	WEIGHT	TIME	NOTES
1			30.0	

© 2020. Candice McField Fitness, LLC. All rights reserved. No part of this publication may be reproduced, distributed, or transmitted in any form, without prior written permission of Candice McField Fitness, LLC. User represents that he/she has consulted with a Physician regarding User's potential use of this workout, prior to beginning the workout, and that the physician consents to User's performance of the workout. The content of the workout and any information otherwise obtained by user through the workout is provided for information purposes only and User uses such information and content AT THE VOLUNTARY, SOLE RISK OF THE USER. USER RELEASES AND RELIEVES, AND AGREES TO RELEASE AND RELIEVE, CANDICE MCFIELD FITNESS, LLC. AND LAUNCHCRATE PUBLISHING, LLC. OF ANY AND ALL LIABILITY FOR ANY INJURIES, CLAIMS OR DAMAGES ARISING OUT OF USER'S USE OF THE SERVICE.

As For Me and My Body

Foam Roller
Candice McField Fitness

| 1 set per exercise | 30 seconds per set | 60 seconds rest between sets |

Equipment: Foam Roller

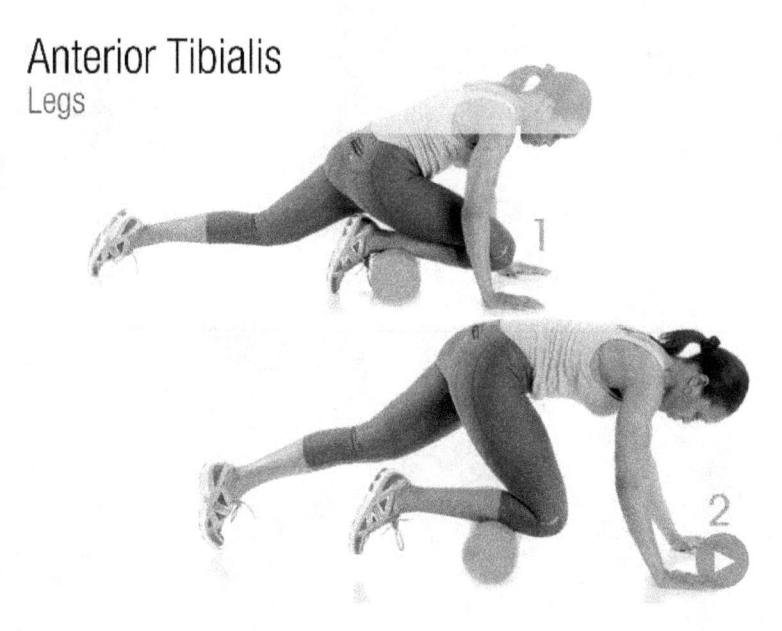

Anterior Tibialis
Legs

scan the code to view a video of the workout

- Position yourself on your hands and knees with the roller under one ankle.
1. Bring one knee into your chest as you support your body on your hands with your ankle on the roller.
2. Rolling up from your ankle to your knee, push back as you straighten your leg.
- Roll back down your shin, keeping your other leg raised throughout.
- Complete all reps on one side before switching to the other side.

#	REPS	WEIGHT	TIME	NOTES
1			30.0	

© 2020. Candice McField Fitness, LLC. All rights reserved. No part of this publication may be reproduced, distributed, or transmitted in any form, without prior written permission of Candice McField Fitness, LLC. User represents that he/she has consulted with a Physician regarding User's potential use of this workout, prior to beginning the workout, and that the physician consents to User's performance of the workout. The content of the workout and any information otherwise obtained by user through the workout is provided for information purposes only and User uses such information and content AT THE VOLUNTARY, SOLE RISK OF THE USER. USER RELEASES AND RELIEVES, AND AGREES TO RELEASE AND RELIEVE, CANDICE MCFIELD FITNESS, LLC. AND LAUNCHCRATE PUBLISHING, LLC. OF ANY AND ALL LIABILITY FOR ANY INJURIES, CLAIMS OR DAMAGES ARISING OUT OF USER'S USE OF THE SERVICE.

Day 19 - Range of Motion

Foam Roller
Candice McField Fitness

1 set	30 seconds	60 seconds
per exercise	per set	rest between sets

Equipment: Foam Roller

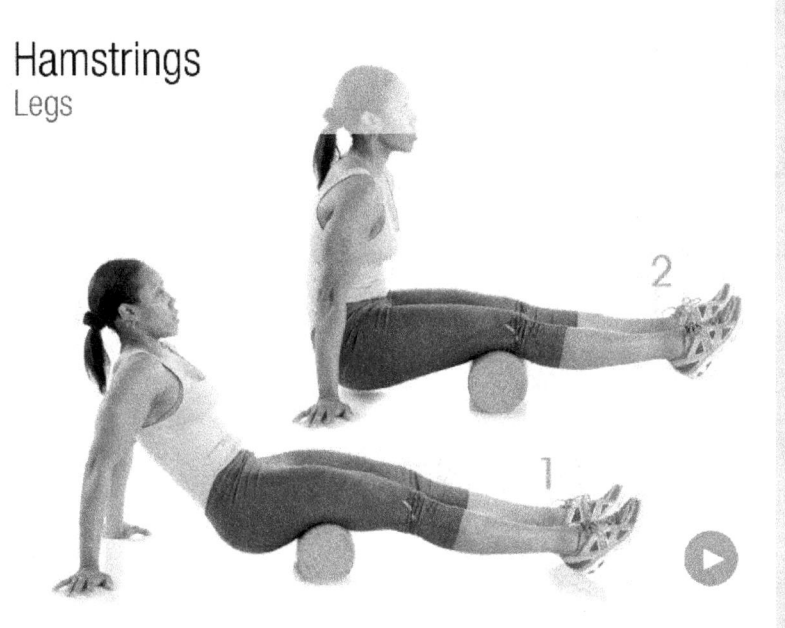

Hamstrings
Legs

1. Sit with a roller under the top of your hamstrings, legs straight, and your hands behind your glutes.
2. Pull your body towards your hands, rolling down along your hamstrings to the back of your knees.
- Push your body back away from your hands, rolling up from your knees to your glutes.

scan the code to view a video of the workout

#	REPS	WEIGHT	TIME	NOTES
1			30.0	

© 2020. Candice McField Fitness, LLC. All rights reserved. No part of this publication may be reproduced, distributed, or transmitted in any form, without prior written permission of Candice McField Fitness, LLC. User represents that he/she has consulted with a Physician regarding User's potential use of this workout, prior to beginning the workout, and that the physician consents to User's performance of the workout. The content of the workout and any information otherwise obtained by user through the workout is provided for information purposes only and User uses such information and content AT THE VOLUNTARY, SOLE RISK OF THE USER. USER RELEASES AND RELIEVES, AND AGREES TO RELEASE AND RELIEVE, CANDICE MCFIELD FITNESS, LLC. AND LAUNCHCRATE PUBLISHING, LLC. OF ANY AND ALL LIABILITY FOR ANY INJURIES, CLAIMS OR DAMAGES ARISING OUT OF USER'S USE OF THE SERVICE.

Foam Roller
Candice McField Fitness

1 set	30 seconds	60 seconds
per exercise	per set	rest between sets

Equipment: Foam Roller

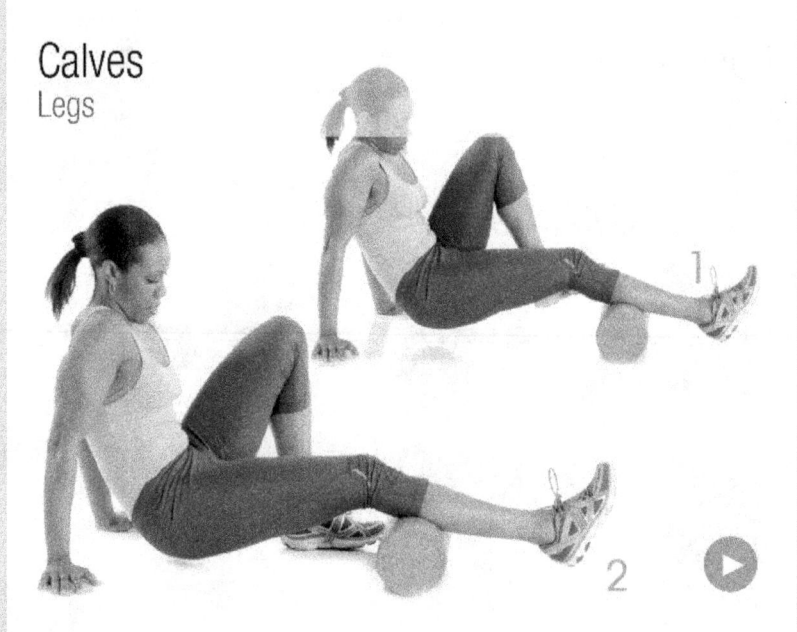

Calves
Legs

scan the code to view a video of the workout

- Sit with your legs extended, a roller under your ankles, and your hands behind your glutes.
1. Raise your hips off the floor as you raise one ankle off the roller, supporting your body on your hands.
2. Roll up and down your calf from your ankle to your knee, pushing your body away with your hands.
- Complete all reps on one side before switching to the other side.

#	REPS	WEIGHT	TIME	NOTES
1			30.0	

© 2020. Candice McField Fitness, LLC. All rights reserved. No part of this publication may be reproduced, distributed, or transmitted in any form, without prior written permission of Candice McField Fitness, LLC. User represents that he/she has consulted with a Physician regarding User's potential use of this workout, prior to beginning the workout, and that the physician consents to User's performance of the workout. The content of the workout and any information otherwise obtained by user through the workout is provided for information purposes only and User uses such information and content AT THE VOLUNTARY, SOLE RISK OF THE USER. USER RELEASES AND RELIEVES, AND AGREES TO RELEASE AND RELIEVE, CANDICE MCFIELD FITNESS, LLC. AND LAUNCHCRATE PUBLISHING, LLC. OF ANY AND ALL LIABILITY FOR ANY INJURIES, CLAIMS OR DAMAGES ARISING OUT OF USER'S USE OF THE SERVICE.

Day 19 - Range of Motion

Foam Roller
Candice McField Fitness

1 set	30 seconds	60 seconds
per exercise	per set	rest between sets

Equipment: Foam Roller

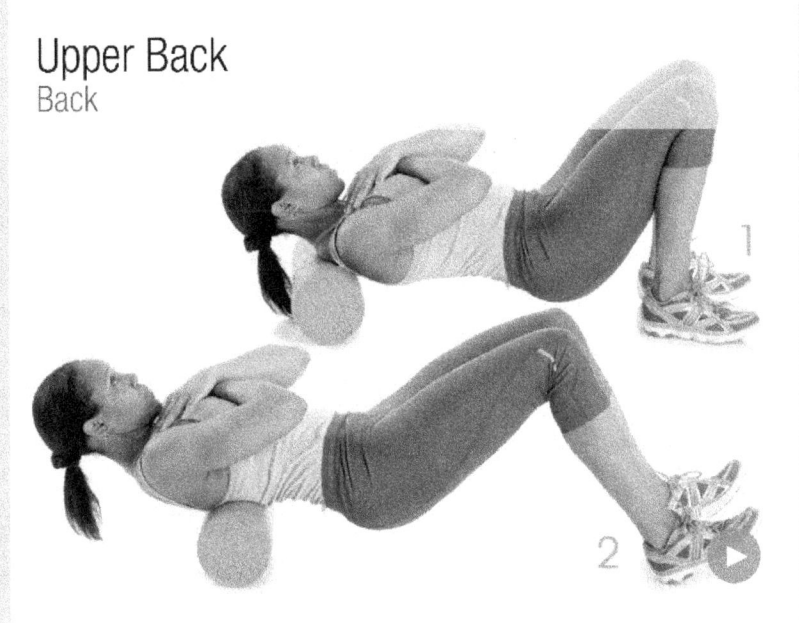

Upper Back
Back

1. Lie with your upper back on a roller with your hands across your chest, knees bent, and feet flat.
2. Roll down from your upper back to your mid back.
- Then roll up from your mid back to your upper back and repeat.

scan the code to view a video of the workout

#	REPS	WEIGHT	TIME	NOTES
1			30.0	

© 2020. Candice McField Fitness, LLC. All rights reserved. No part of this publication may be reproduced, distributed, or transmitted in any form, without prior written permission of Candice McField Fitness, LLC. User represents that he/she has consulted with a Physician regarding User's potential use of this workout, prior to beginning the workout, and that the physician consents to User's performance of the workout. The content of the workout and any information otherwise obtained by user through the workout is provided for information purposes only and User uses such information and content AT THE VOLUNTARY, SOLE RISK OF THE USER. USER RELEASES AND RELIEVES, AND AGREES TO RELEASE AND RELIEVE, CANDICE MCFIELD FITNESS, LLC. AND LAUNCHCRATE PUBLISHING, LLC. OF ANY AND ALL LIABILITY FOR ANY INJURIES, CLAIMS OR DAMAGES ARISING OUT OF USER'S USE OF THE SERVICE.

Foam Roller
Candice McField Fitness

| 1 set per exercise | 30 seconds per set | 60 seconds rest between sets |

Equipment: Foam Roller

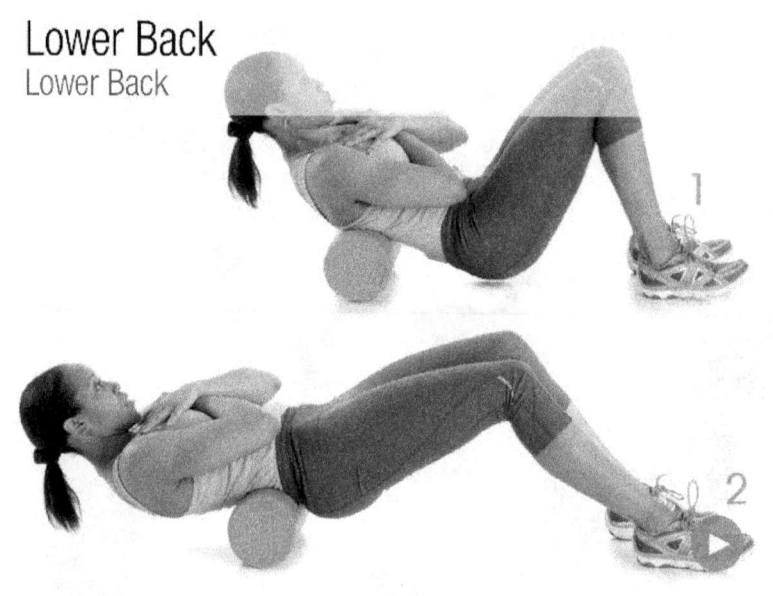

Lower Back
Lower Back

1. Lie with a roller at your mid-back with knees bent, and your feet flat.
2. Push forward, rolling down from your mid-back to your glutes.
- Pull back, rolling up from your glutes to your mid-back.

scan the code to view a video of the workout

#	REPS	WEIGHT	TIME	NOTES
1			30.0	

© 2020. Candice McField Fitness, LLC. All rights reserved. No part of this publication may be reproduced, distributed, or transmitted in any form, without prior written permission of Candice McField Fitness, LLC. User represents that he/she has consulted with a Physician regarding User's potential use of this workout, prior to beginning the workout, and that the physician consents to User's performance of the workout. The content of the workout and any information otherwise obtained by user through the workout is provided for information purposes only and User uses such information and content AT THE VOLUNTARY, SOLE RISK OF THE USER. USER RELEASES AND RELIEVES, AND AGREES TO RELEASE AND RELIEVE, CANDICE MCFIELD FITNESS, LLC. AND LAUNCHCRATE PUBLISHING, LLC. OF ANY AND ALL LIABILITY FOR ANY INJURIES, CLAIMS OR DAMAGES ARISING OUT OF USER'S USE OF THE SERVICE.

Day 19 - Range of Motion

Foam Roller
Candice McField Fitness

1 set per exercise | **30 seconds** per set | **60 seconds** rest between sets

Equipment: Foam Roller

Quadriceps
Legs

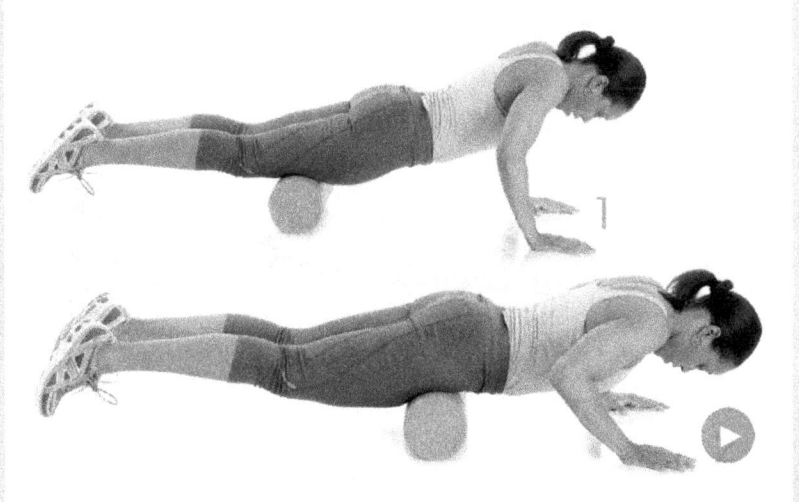

1. Lie face down, place a roller just above your knees and under your lower thighs.
2. Push away and roll from your knees to your mid-thighs.
- Pull back, rolling down to the top of your knees.

scan the code to view a video of the workout

#	REPS	WEIGHT	TIME	NOTES
1			30.0	

© 2020. Candice McField Fitness, LLC. All rights reserved. No part of this publication may be reproduced, distributed, or transmitted in any form, without prior written permission of Candice McField Fitness, LLC. User represents that he/she has consulted with a Physician regarding User's potential use of this workout, prior to beginning the workout, and that the physician consents to User's performance of the workout. The content of the workout and any information otherwise obtained by user through the workout is provided for information purposes only and User uses such information and content AT THE VOLUNTARY, SOLE RISK OF THE USER. USER RELEASES AND RELIEVES, AND AGREES TO RELEASE AND RELIEVE, CANDICE MCFIELD FITNESS, LLC. AND LAUNCHCRATE PUBLISHING, LLC. OF ANY AND ALL LIABILITY FOR ANY INJURIES, CLAIMS OR DAMAGES ARISING OUT OF USER'S USE OF THE SERVICE.

Foam Roller
Candice McField Fitness

1 set	30 seconds	60 seconds
per exercise	per set	rest between sets

Equipment: Foam Roller

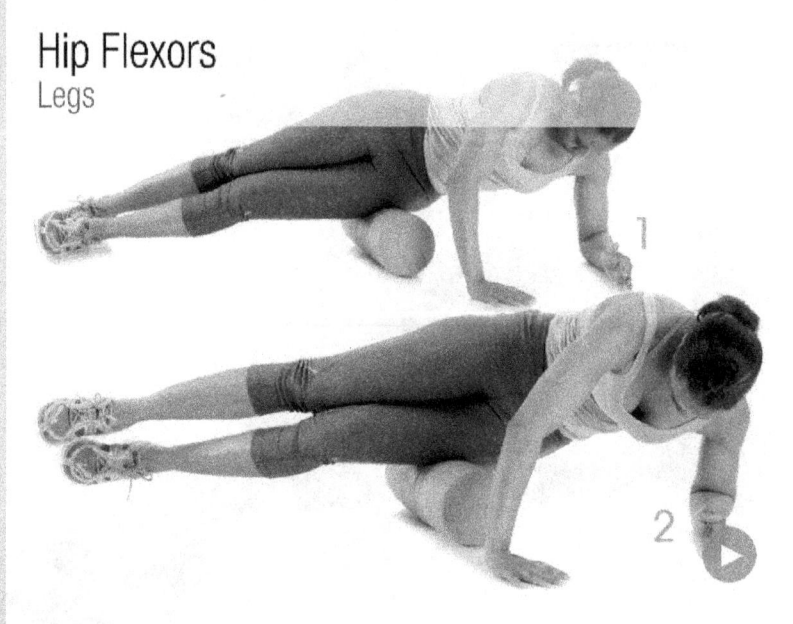

Hip Flexors
Legs

scan the code to view a video of the workout

1. Lie on your side with a roller at hip level. Extend your leg on the roller off the floor and bend your other leg 90-degrees.
2. Roll up and down your leg from the top of your hip to your mid-quad.
- Complete all reps on one side before switching to the other side.

#	REPS	WEIGHT	TIME	NOTES
1			30.0	

© 2020. Candice McField Fitness, LLC. All rights reserved. No part of this publication may be reproduced, distributed, or transmitted in any form, without prior written permission of Candice McField Fitness, LLC. User represents that he/she has consulted with a Physician regarding User's potential use of this workout, prior to beginning the workout, and that the physician consents to User's performance of the workout. The content of the workout and any information otherwise obtained by user through the workout is provided for information purposes only and User uses such information and content AT THE VOLUNTARY, SOLE RISK OF THE USER. USER RELEASES AND RELIEVES, AND AGREES TO RELEASE AND RELIEVE, CANDICE MCFIELD FITNESS, LLC. AND LAUNCHCRATE PUBLISHING, LLC. OF ANY AND ALL LIABILITY FOR ANY INJURIES, CLAIMS OR DAMAGES ARISING OUT OF USER'S USE OF THE SERVICE.

Day 19 - Range of Motion

Foam Roller
Candice McField Fitness

| 1 set per exercise | 30 seconds per set | 60 seconds rest between sets |

Equipment: Foam Roller

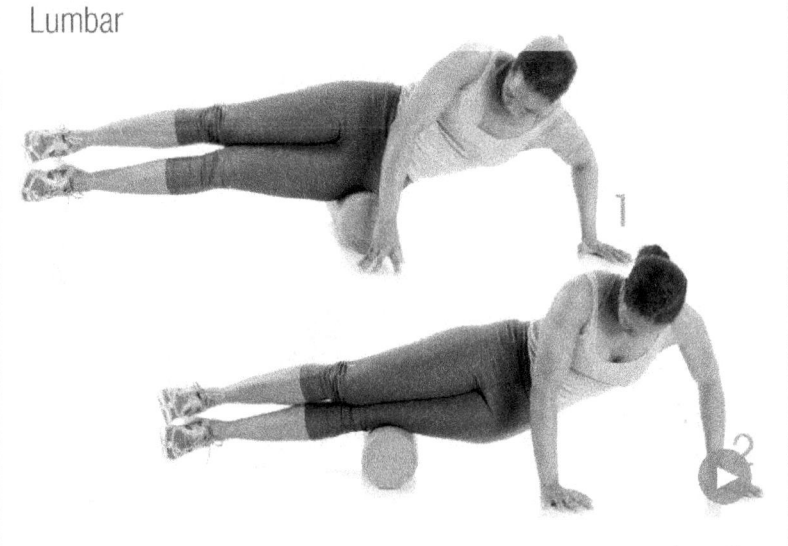

IT Band
Lumbar

scan the code to view a video of the workout

1. Lie on your side with a roller under your hip, feet off the floor and hands on the floor.
2. Draw your body towards your arms, rolling down along the side of your thigh from your hip to the top of your knee.
- Push away rolling back up the side of your thigh from your knee to your hip.
- Complete all reps on one side before switching to the other side.

#	REPS	WEIGHT	TIME	NOTES
1			30.0	

© 2020. Candice McField Fitness, LLC. All rights reserved. No part of this publication may be reproduced, distributed, or transmitted in any form, without prior written permission of Candice McField Fitness, LLC. User represents that he/she has consulted with a Physician regarding User's potential use of this workout, prior to beginning the workout, and that the physician consents to User's performance of the workout. The content of the workout and any information otherwise obtained by user through the workout is provided for information purposes only and User uses such information and content AT THE VOLUNTARY, SOLE RISK OF THE USER. USER RELEASES AND RELIEVES, AND AGREES TO RELEASE AND RELIEVE, CANDICE MCFIELD FITNESS, LLC. AND LAUNCHCRATE PUBLISHING, LLC. OF ANY AND ALL LIABILITY FOR ANY INJURIES, CLAIMS OR DAMAGES ARISING OUT OF USER'S USE OF THE SERVICE.

As For Me and My Body

Foam Roller
Candice McField Fitness

1 set	30 seconds	60 seconds
per exercise	per set	rest between sets

Equipment: Foam Roller

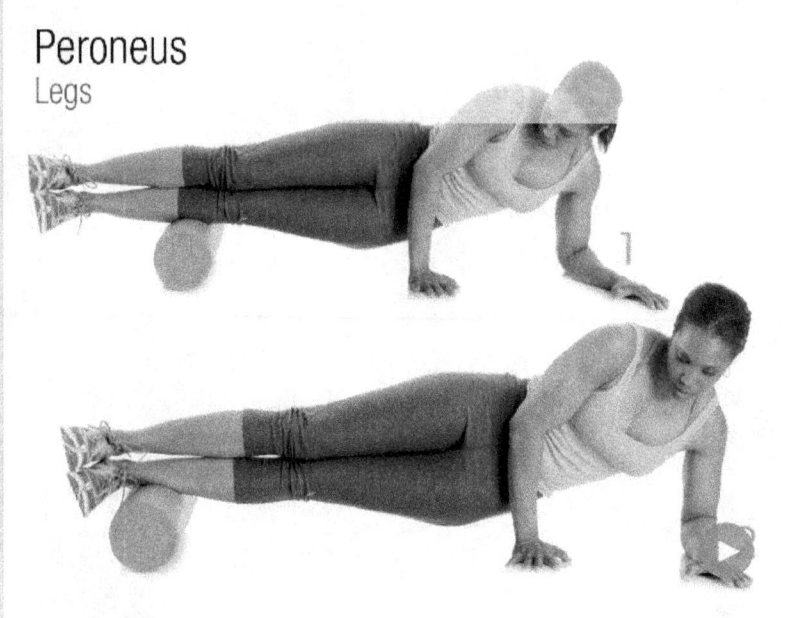

Peroneus
Legs

scan the code to view a video of the workout

1. Lie on your side, placing a roller under the side of your bottom shin.
2. Pull your body towards your forearm, rolling down the side of your shin, from your knee to your ankle.
- Push away, rolling back up the side of your shin to your knee.
- Complete all reps on one side before switching to the other side.

#	REPS	WEIGHT	TIME	NOTES
1			30.0	

© 2020. Candice McField Fitness, LLC. All rights reserved. No part of this publication may be reproduced, distributed, or transmitted in any form, without prior written permission of Candice McField Fitness, LLC. User represents that he/she has consulted with a Physician regarding User's potential use of this workout, prior to beginning the workout, and that the physician consents to User's performance of the workout. The content of the workout and any information otherwise obtained by user through the workout is provided for information purposes only and User uses such information and content AT THE VOLUNTARY, SOLE RISK OF THE USER. USER RELEASES AND RELIEVES, AND AGREES TO RELEASE AND RELIEVE, CANDICE MCFIELD FITNESS, LLC. AND LAUNCHCRATE PUBLISHING, LLC. OF ANY AND ALL LIABILITY FOR ANY INJURIES, CLAIMS OR DAMAGES ARISING OUT OF USER'S USE OF THE SERVICE.

Day 19 - Range of Motion

Day 19
Unlocking My Optimal Performance

Moment of Truth: Flexibility, is often the most neglected component of physical fitness.

Quote to Remember: "True flexibility can be achieved only when all muscles are uniformly developed."
— Joseph H. Pilates

Challenge to Implement: Commit to stretching 10 minutes daily. One suggestion is to make it a part of your morning, night, or other daily routine.

Soli Deo Gloria and *Arise!*®

Candice

The Importance of Flexibility

I commit to stretch daily for 10 minutes in the: morning, afternoon, or at night (circle one)

Day 18

Core
Your Foundation

Spiritually, our core is Christ, as I mentioned on Day 17. Often, we look to ourselves to fix things, solve problems, and for strength. Even worse, we often pat ourselves on the back to congratulate our efforts, thinking "we" did this. Yet, the entire time we have forgotten that He did it. He fixed it. He solved it. He was our strength carrying us through. We are simply stewards, hence, it is never us! Christ is our core, our foundation, our source of being, and our strength.

It is when we begin to rely on personal pronouns, I, that we begin to fall face down. In the song, *Weak*, by Dillon Chase, he has a line that epitomizes this principal. The lyrics are:

> *"But humility really it is a gem*
> *Where do I begin*
> *Oh, I remember now why I am so down*
> *And the answer is found in personal pronouns*
> *Looking to I to fly, fall face down*
> *Thinking I can ride this whole thing out."*

My pastor explained humility beautifully when speaking on Philippians 2:3-5. He emphasized, "Humility is **not** thinking less of yourself, it is thinking not of yourself!" Jesus displayed the ultimate example of humility, so let us always remember to never focus on the personal pronoun, I.

Regarding fitness, having a strong core is essential for exercise performance and enjoyment. Our core, the midsection of our body, needs to be solid, strong, and the musculature needs to be able to stabilize spinal and pelvic positioning, as well as contract dynamically because it is the key link that connects movements between the upper and lower body.

Day 17
Unlocking My Optimal Performance

Moment of Truth: Christ is our core, our foundation, our source of being, and our strength.

Verse to Remember: *"Don't be selfish; don't try to impress others. Be humble, thinking of others as better than yourselves."*
Philippians 2:3 (NLT)

Challenge to Implement: *Recall a time you looked to yourself and not to God for guidance, strength, and solutions. What was the outcome? How different do you think it may have been if Christ was guiding you, rather than yourself?*

Soli Deo Gloria and *Arise!*®

Candice

The body's core is the origin or insertion point for nearly 30 muscles in the abdomen, low back, pelvis, and hips. These muscles transfer force to and from the upper and lower extremities.

If you view the body as a chain, it is only as strong as its

Day 18 - Core - Your Foundation

weakest link. If you have strong legs and arms, but an undeveloped lower torso or trunk, force cannot efficiently be transferred between the upper and lower body. This is because your midsection lacks the strength to stabilize the lower torso during movement. In other words, the body needs a strong foundation from which to direct efforts so energy that is created for movements ends up being a part of that movement, rather than wasted. Misdirected energy is not harmless; it can lead to poor performance and injury. Essentially, our core is our foundation and the body needs a strong foundation.

Benefits of a Strong Core

Spares the spine from damage	Avoid injury
Directs effort correctly	Improves exercise performance
Avoid poor performance	Improves exercise enjoyment
Creates a stable and mobile lower back	

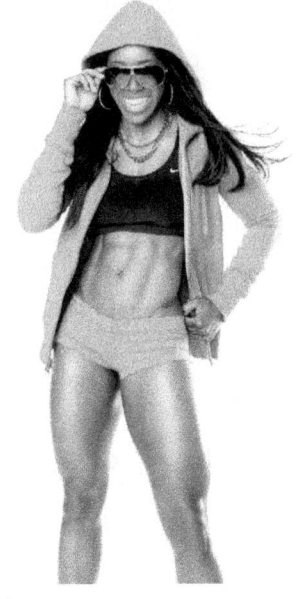

A huge misconception about core training is that one needs to do hundreds of reps to create washboard abs. This is a myth, and far from the truth. First, the abdominals are one of the last muscle groups to show definition when trying to lose body fat. Secondly, cardio and nutrition play huge roles in being able to 'see' your abs. You can do hundreds of ab exercises daily and never see your abs if you do not burn off the fat that is overlaying your ab muscles! Hence, the saying that abs are made in the kitchen through clean eating is very true. In addition, one must also do cardio and strength training. Adequate core training should be performed four times each week. For instance, I train my core on Mondays, Tuesdays, Thursdays, and Fridays and I do not perform hundreds of reps. My ab routine consists of 6 exercises at 12 reps per exercise. Afterwards, I perform two more core exercises for 2 sets of 20 reps.

Give my routine a try. Enjoy!

Day 18 – Core – Your Foundation

Ab Routine
Candice McField Fitness

| 2 sets per exercise | 12 reps per set | 60 seconds rest between sets |

Equipment: none required

Leg Raise Mini

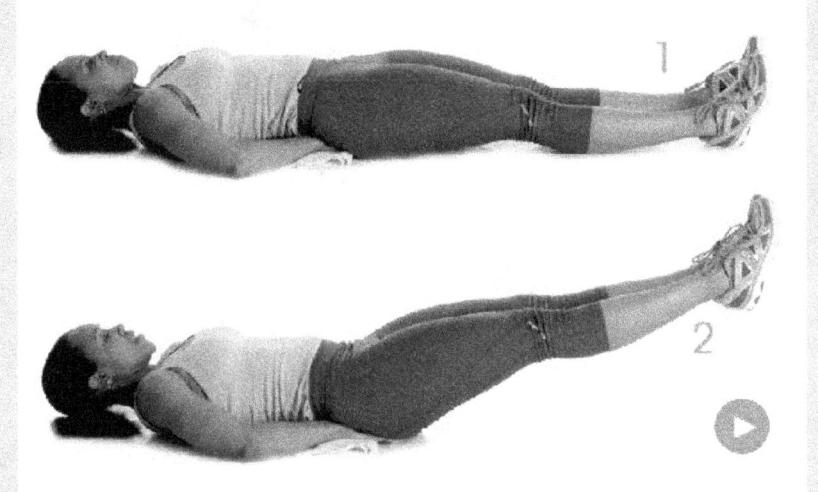

1. Lie on your back with your legs straight and your hands under your glutes.
2. Raise your legs straight up, approximately 1 foot off the floor.
- Slowly lower your legs, keeping your upper body stable and your legs straight throughout.

scan the code to view a video of the workout

#	REPS	WEIGHT	TIME	NOTES
1	12		0.0	
2	12			

© 2020. Candice McField Fitness, LLC. All rights reserved. No part of this publication may be reproduced, distributed, or transmitted in any form, without prior written permission of Candice McField Fitness, LLC. User represents that he/she has consulted with a Physician regarding User's potential use of this workout, prior to beginning the workout, and that the physician consents to User's performance of the workout. The content of the workout and any information otherwise obtained by user through the workout is provided for information purposes only and User uses such information and content AT THE VOLUNTARY, SOLE RISK OF THE USER. USER RELEASES AND RELIEVES, AND AGREES TO RELEASE AND RELIEVE, CANDICE MCFIELD FITNESS, LLC. AND LAUNCHCRATE PUBLISHING, LLC. OF ANY AND ALL LIABILITY FOR ANY INJURIES, CLAIMS OR DAMAGES ARISING OUT OF USER'S USE OF THE SERVICE.

Ab Routine
Candice McField Fitness

| 2 sets per exercise | 12 reps per set | 60 seconds rest between sets |

Equipment: none required

Crunch

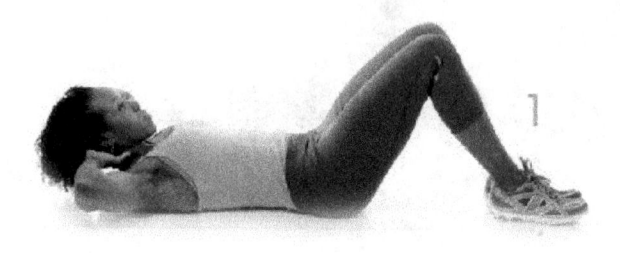

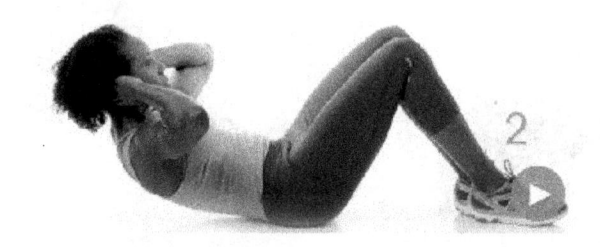

scan the code to view a video of the workout

1. Lie on your back with your knees bent and feet flat. Place your hands behind your head.
2. Lift your head and shoulders off the floor, keeping your feet flat.
- Lower your head and shoulders and repeat.
- Do not pull your head up with your hands.

#	REPS	WEIGHT	TIME	NOTES
1	12		0.0	
2	12			

© 2020. Candice McField Fitness, LLC. All rights reserved. No part of this publication may be reproduced, distributed, or transmitted in any form, without prior written permission of Candice McField Fitness, LLC. User represents that he/she has consulted with a Physician regarding User's potential use of this workout, prior to beginning the workout, and that the physician consents to User's performance of the workout. The content of the workout and any information otherwise obtained by user through the workout is provided for information purposes only and User uses such information and content AT THE VOLUNTARY, SOLE RISK OF THE USER. USER RELEASES AND RELIEVES, AND AGREES TO RELEASE AND RELIEVE, CANDICE MCFIELD FITNESS, LLC. AND LAUNCHCRATE PUBLISHING, LLC. OF ANY AND ALL LIABILITY FOR ANY INJURIES, CLAIMS OR DAMAGES ARISING OUT OF USER'S USE OF THE SERVICE.

Day 18 - Core - Your Foundation

Ab Routine
Candice McField Fitness

2 sets per exercise
12 reps per set
60 seconds rest between sets

Equipment: none required

Side Abs

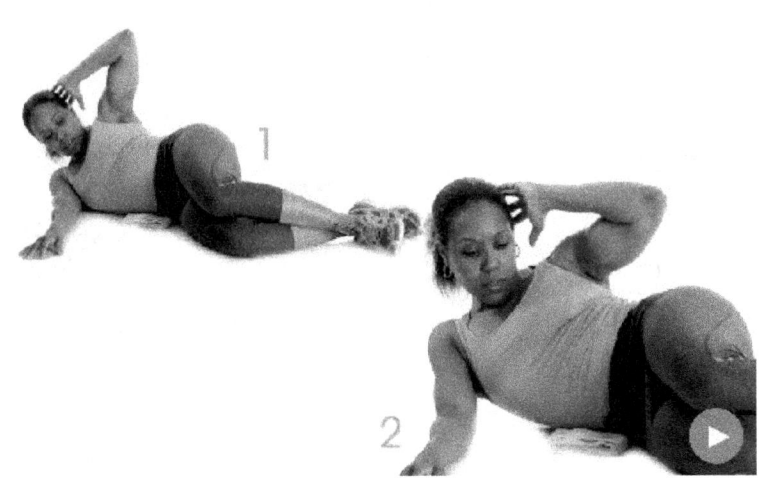

scan the code to view a video of the workout

1. Lie on your side with your lower body twisted to one side, knees bent, one arm extended, and one hand placed behind your head. Align the elbow of your top arm directly over your hip.
2. Lift your head and shoulders off the floor, keeping your lower body stable.
- Lower your head and shoulders and repeat.

#	REPS	WEIGHT	TIME	NOTES
1	12		0.0	
2	12			

© 2020. Candice McField Fitness, LLC. All rights reserved. No part of this publication may be reproduced, distributed, or transmitted in any form, without prior written permission of Candice McField Fitness, LLC. User represents that he/she has consulted with a Physician regarding User's potential use of this workout, prior to beginning the workout, and that the physician consents to User's performance of the workout. The content of the workout and any information otherwise obtained by user through the workout is provided for information purposes only and User uses such information and content AT THE VOLUNTARY, SOLE RISK OF THE USER. USER RELEASES AND RELIEVES, AND AGREES TO RELEASE AND RELIEVE, CANDICE MCFIELD FITNESS, LLC. AND LAUNCHCRATE PUBLISHING, LLC. OF ANY AND ALL LIABILITY FOR ANY INJURIES, CLAIMS OR DAMAGES ARISING OUT OF USER'S USE OF THE SERVICE.

Ab Routine
Candice McField Fitness

2 sets per exercise | **12 reps** per set | **60 seconds** rest between sets

Equipment: none required

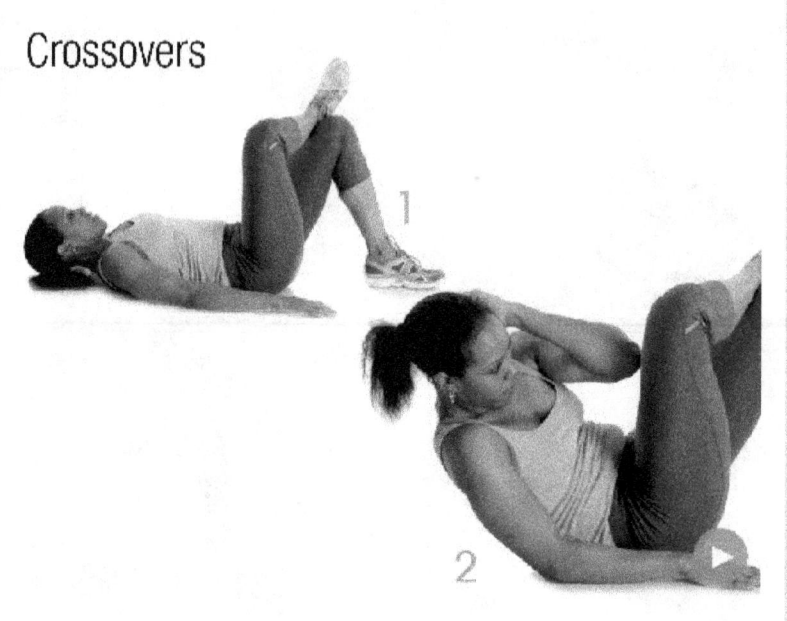

Crossovers

scan the code to view a video of the workout

1. Lie on your back with one foot flat on the floor, one knee bent and your other foot on top of this knee. Place your hands to the sides of your head.
2. Lift your head and shoulders off the floor and twist your torso towards the raised knee.
- Lower your head and shoulders and repeat.
- Complete all reps on one side before switching to the other side.

#	REPS	WEIGHT	TIME	NOTES
1	12		0.0	
2	12			

© 2020. Candice McField Fitness, LLC. All rights reserved. No part of this publication may be reproduced, distributed, or transmitted in any form, without prior written permission of Candice McField Fitness, LLC. User represents that he/she has consulted with a Physician regarding User's potential use of this workout, prior to beginning the workout, and that the physician consents to User's performance of the workout. The content of the workout and any information otherwise obtained by user through the workout is provided for information purposes only and User uses such information and content AT THE VOLUNTARY, SOLE RISK OF THE USER. USER RELEASES AND RELIEVES, AND AGREES TO RELEASE AND RELIEVE, CANDICE MCFIELD FITNESS, LLC. AND LAUNCHCRATE PUBLISHING, LLC. OF ANY AND ALL LIABILITY FOR ANY INJURIES, CLAIMS OR DAMAGES ARISING OUT OF USER'S USE OF THE SERVICE.

Day 18 - Core - Your Foundation

Ab Routine
Candice McField Fitness

| 2 sets per exercise | 12 reps per set | 60 seconds rest between sets |

Equipment: none required

Sit Up 2

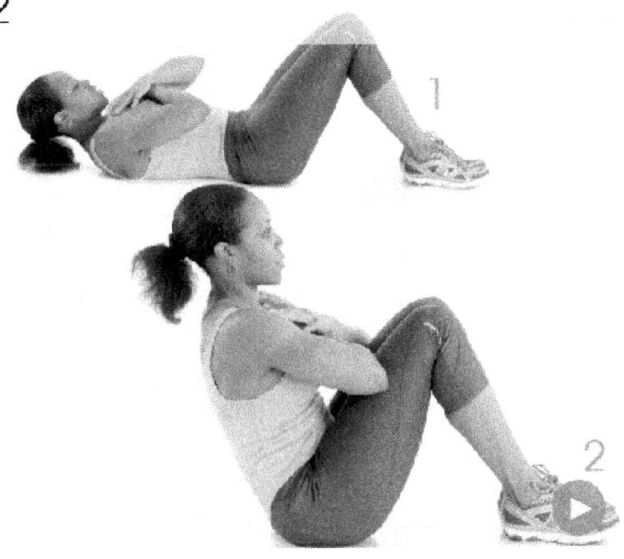

scan the code to view a video of the workout

1. Lie on your back, knees bent and feet flat with your hands crossed over your chest.
2. Lift your upper body off the floor, bringing your chest to your knees.
- Keep your feet flat, knees bent, and do not pull yourself up with momentum. Focus on using your abdominals.
- Lower your upper body to the floor and repeat.

#	REPS	WEIGHT	TIME	NOTES
1	12		0.0	
2	12			

© 2020. Candice McField Fitness, LLC. All rights reserved. No part of this publication may be reproduced, distributed, or transmitted in any form, without prior written permission of Candice McField Fitness, LLC. User represents that he/she has consulted with a Physician regarding User's potential use of this workout, prior to beginning the workout, and that the physician consents to User's performance of the workout. The content of the workout and any information otherwise obtained by user through the workout is provided for information purposes only and User uses such information and content AT THE VOLUNTARY, SOLE RISK OF THE USER. USER RELEASES AND RELIEVES, AND AGREES TO RELEASE AND RELIEVE, CANDICE MCFIELD FITNESS, LLC. AND LAUNCHCRATE PUBLISHING, LLC. OF ANY AND ALL LIABILITY FOR ANY INJURIES, CLAIMS OR DAMAGES ARISING OUT OF USER'S USE OF THE SERVICE.

Ab Routine
Candice McField Fitness

2 sets per exercise
12 reps per set
60 seconds rest between sets

Equipment: none required

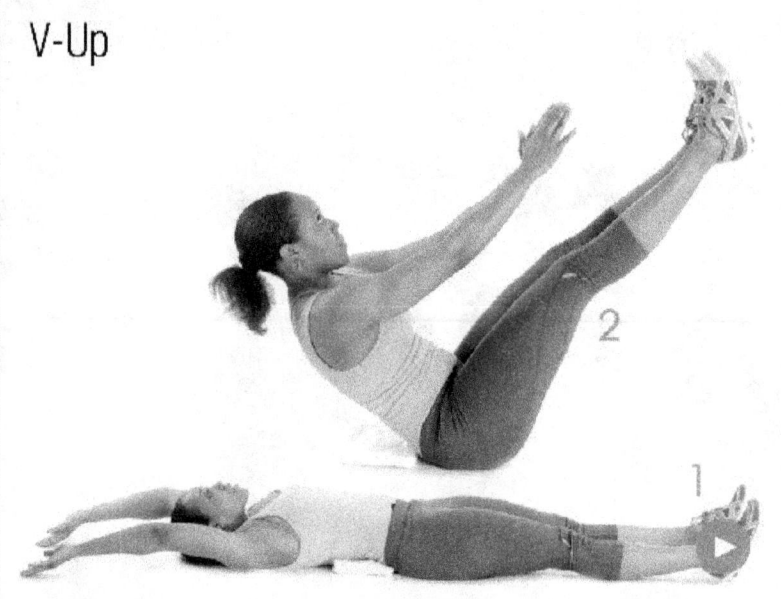

V-Up

1. Lie on your back with your legs straight and with your arms stretched out overhead.
2. Raise your legs straight up as you lift your upper body off the floor and reach your hands towards your feet.
- Slowly lower your upper body and legs back to the floor and repeat.

scan the code to view a video of the workout

#	REPS	WEIGHT	TIME	NOTES
1	12		0.0	
2	12			

© 2020. Candice McField Fitness, LLC. All rights reserved. No part of this publication may be reproduced, distributed, or transmitted in any form, without prior written permission of Candice McField Fitness, LLC. User represents that he/she has consulted with a Physician regarding User's potential use of this workout, prior to beginning the workout, and that the physician consents to User's performance of the workout. The content of the workout and any information otherwise obtained by user through the workout is provided for information purposes only and User uses such information and content AT THE VOLUNTARY, SOLE RISK OF THE USER. USER RELEASES AND RELIEVES, AND AGREES TO RELEASE AND RELIEVE, CANDICE MCFIELD FITNESS, LLC. AND LAUNCHCRATE PUBLISHING, LLC. OF ANY AND ALL LIABILITY FOR ANY INJURIES, CLAIMS OR DAMAGES ARISING OUT OF USER'S USE OF THE SERVICE.

Day 18 - Core - Your Foundation

Day 18

Unlocking My Optimal Performance

Moment of Truth: A huge misconception about core training is that one needs to do hundreds of reps to create washboard abs.

Quote to Remember: "You can train and train until you are blue in the face, but you've got to diet, you've got to have that leanness because if you are not lean, your abs won't show."
- Henry Cavill

Challenge to Implement: Rate the condition of your core. Next, determine if you are getting in an adequate amount of core exercise. Lastly, commit to do ing core four times per week.

Soli Deo Gloria and *Arise!*®

Candice

The Importance of Core

I feel my current core level and strength is:
below average, average, or above average

I currently work my core:
0, 1, 2, 3, 4, 5, 6, or 7 times per week

Going forward, I will work my core on these days of the week: Monday, Tuesday, Wednesday, Thursday, Friday, Saturday, Sunday

Day 19

Relapse Prevention

I was in middle school when my grandmother told me to keep a journal. I did not question why she wanted me to begin writing things down, I simply accepted the challenge. I am beyond grateful because her suggestion is one of the most practical and meaningful things in my life. I now have a collection of thoughts dating back to middle school that allowed me to remember significant aspects of my life. I can see how far I have come, recall the goodness of God's grace and mercy, and understand His personal, ever presence in my life.

I love reading Joshua 4:4-23, that depicts when the Israelites built a memorial to remember the crossing of the Jordan River.

> "So Joshua called together the twelve men he had chosen one from each of the tribes of Israel. He told them, 'Go into the middle of the Jordan, in front of the Ark of the Lord your God. Each of you must pick up one stone and carry it out on your shoulder twelve stones in all, one for each of the twelve tribes of Israel. We will use these stones to build a memorial. In the future your children will ask you, 'What do these stones mean?' Then you can tell them, 'They remind us that the Jordan River stopped flowing

when the Ark of the Lord's Covenant went across...This is where the Israelites crossed the Jordan on dry ground.' For the Lord your God dried up the river right before your eyes, and he kept it dry until you were all across, just as he did at the Red Sea when he dried it up until we had all crossed over."

To reduce our lapses in our Christian walk, we should now still build memorials in our heart, mind, soul, and physical world to help us remember how God has brought us through!

Day 19
Unlocking My Optimal Performance

Moment of Truth: Building memorials in our heart, mind, soul, and physical world, helps us remember how God has brought us through!

Verse to Remember: "We will use these stones to build a memorial. In the future your children will ask you, 'What do these stones mean?' Then you can tell them, 'They remind us that the Jordan River stopped flowing when the Ark of the Lord's Covenant went across."

Joshua 4:6-7 (NLT)

Challenge to Implement: Begin keeping a spiritual journal in order to reflect on the past and how God has always brought you through. If you already keep one, re read your last year of entries and simply give thanks for His continually presence in your life.

Soli Deo Gloria and *Arise!*®

Candice

Day 19 - Relapse Prevention

WEIGHT LOSS

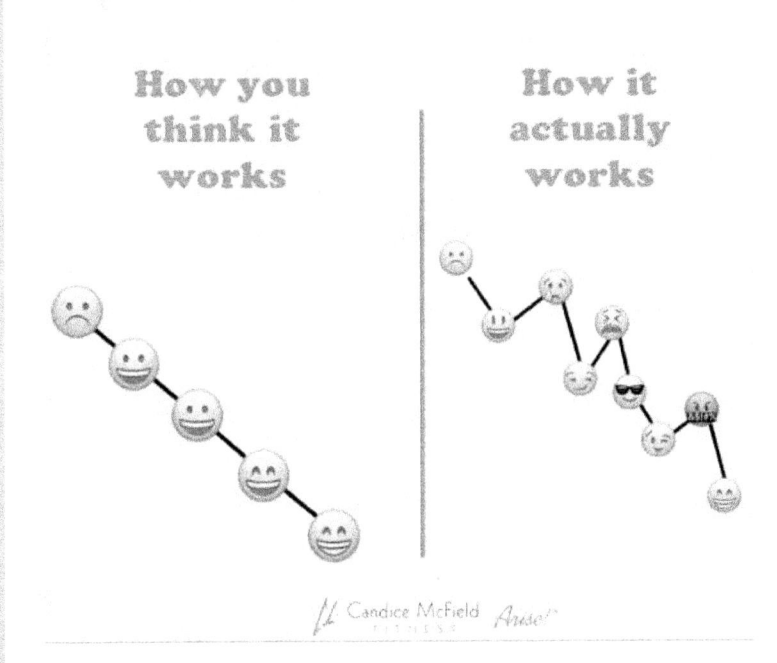

How you think it works

How it actually works

Candice McField

During your health and fitness journey, you may experience some frustration or disappointment in your progress. You may perceive yourself as failing and be ready to give up. Fluctuations during your health and fitness journey are normal. In fact, throughout this process there are going to be many peaks and valleys. As you experience those peaks and valleys, your key focus must remain on your long--term goals. In other words, if you were to graph your progress overtime, it is common to see a zig-zag line filled with high and lows, yet, overtime it indicates you are progressing.

Valleys, also known as lapses during training, should be viewed as opportunities for fine-tuning, not failure. Your valleys are indicators to start another phase of active management. When you shift your focus to actively manage and fine-tune your activities during these times, you avoid relapses.

As For Me and My Body

Lapses are normal and should be taken in stride. You may feel disappointed when lapses happen but do not allow yourself to feel guilty or as if you failed. When negative thoughts and emotions overpower our self-control, the domino effect begins, increasing stress and ultimately, leading to relapse.

Think about a baby learning to walk. In the beginning, they fall a lot, sometimes become frustrated, and even need help. Through it all, they never give up and no one would ever tell a baby to stop trying, or that they will never walk. Your fitness journey should be viewed the same way; your long-term goals must outweigh your short--term desires. **Do not give up.**

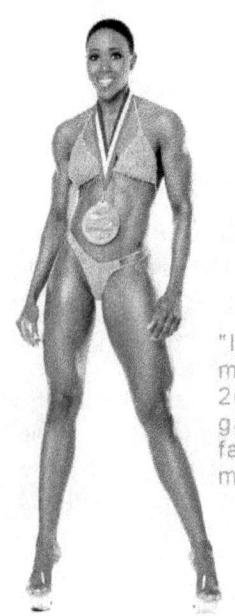

Candice McField
FITNESS

Arise!

Resilience

"I've missed more than 9,000 shots in my career. I've lost almost 300 games. 26 times, I've been trusted to take the game winning shot and missed. I've failed over and over and over again in my life. And that is why I succeed."

~Michael Jordan

Day 19 - Relapse Prevention

Because the vast majority of people face one or more barriers, such as time, finances, prioritizing, scheduling, support issues, etc. it is important to develop strategies before adherence problems arise. Four strategies are:

1. **Increase social support.** The more you increase and maintain social support for exercise, by getting family and friends involved in your journey to some degree, the more likely you are to reach your health and fitness goals.
2. **Become more assertive.** The more assertive you are regarding your progress, concerns, accomplishments, and struggles, the more likely you are to achieve long-term success.
3. **Improve your self-regulation.** The more effective you become at self-regulating your behaviors, schedules, time, and priorities, the more likely you will adhere to your game plan.
4. **Identify high-risk situations.** The more prepared you are at identifying and forming solutions for high-risk situations, the more likely you are to remain physically active during these barriers.

Let's prevent your lapses from turning into relapses!

As For Me and My Body

Day 19
Unlocking My Optimal Performance

Moment of Truth: Lapses during training should be viewed as opportunities for fine tuning, not failure.

Quote to Remember: "I've missed more than 9,000 shots in my career. I've lost almost 300 games. 26 times, I've been trusted to take the game winning shot and missed. I've failed over and over and over again I my life. And that is why I succeed."

— Michael Jordan

Challenge to Implement:
1) Complete the Strategies to Prevent Relapses Worksheet

2) Identify your goal weight, clothes size, etc. Whatever measurement factor(s) are most important to you. Next, identify your relapse prevention goal weight, clothes size, etc. Ex: If your goal weight is 130 pounds you could set your relapse prevention weight at 135 pounds. Hence, if you get back up to 135 pounds that is your signal to tighten up your workout and nutrition regimen.

Soli Deo Gloria and *Arise!*®

Candice

Day 19 - Relapse Prevention

Strategies to Prevent Relapses

The vast majority of people face one or more barriers, such as time, finances, prioritizing, scheduling, support issues, etc. It is important to develop strategies before adherence problems arise.

Step 1: Identify the high-risk situations that most often deter you from being consistent when following a health and fitness regimen:

FINANCES
- ○ Financial constraints

GOALS
- ○ Failure to reach goals
- ○ Unrealistic goals
- ○ Loss interest in keeping records

MYSELF
- ○ Lack of self-motivation
- ○ Lack of confidence in my ability
- ○ Physical injury
- ○ Health concerns/problem

PRIORITIZING & SCHEDULING
- ○ Lack of convenience
- ○ Schedule conflict with other activities
- ○ Schedule conflict with partner

SUPPORT
- ○ Lack of activity partner(s)
- ○ Lack of available childcare
- ○ Goals too challenging

TIME
- ○ Busy home/family schedule
- ○ Busy work schedule

MISCELLANEOUS
- ○ Gym/club environment
- ○ Inclement weather
- ○ Other:
- ○ Insufficient activities or amenities

Step 2: For each identified high-risk situation, devise a coping strategy to overcome the obstacle.

Obstacle	Coping Strategy

Relapse Prevention

Identify your goal weight, clothes size, etc. Whatever measurement factor(s) are most important to you. Next, identify your relapse prevention goal weight, clothes size, etc. Ex: If your goal weight is 130 pounds you could set your relapse prevention weight at 135 pounds. Hence, if you get back up to 135 pounds that is your signal to tighten up your workout and nutrition regimen.

Goal 1

Relapse Prevention Goal

Goal 2

Relapse Prevention Goal

Goal 3

Relapse Prevention Goal

Day 19 - Relapse Prevention

Day 20

Unlock Optimal Performance

In 2013, I took an unforgettable trip with my mom which left me inspired. We were attending my friend's wedding in Guanajuato, Mexico. Before leaving the United States, we had a layover in San Antonio and stayed the evening with family friends. In their house was a decorative sign that read,

> "We all have within our reach the potential to do great things. The difference between the possible and the impossible is sometimes merely perception and attitude. It is the ability to dream beyond ourselves, beyond our own strength and have a faith to believe in the unbelievable. Limitations are the product of the world...possibilities the product of faith. We can expect nothing more than that which we believe possible."

As I mentioned in *Day 11*, we must strive to have unshakable faith, like the Roman officer. Once we realize and implement this concept in our lives, we will dream beyond ourselves, beyond our own strengths, and have faith to believe in the unbelievable. Faith is how we spiritually unlock optimal performance.

On *Day 5*, I wrote about how it was such an honor to read the Bible to my grandmother every evening. In 2012, at the age of 96, God called her home. I was at the hospital the morning of the day she passed. I had the privilege, honor, and opportunity to read to her one last time as her "teacher." After reading the entire chapter of Hebrews 11, The Hall of Faith, I told her, "Granny, soon you will be in the Hall of Faith what a privilege and honor." She transitioned to Heaven that afternoon.

As believers, one of the best and most humble honors we could receive is to be a "Hall of Faith" example for someone or to have someone place us in their personal Hall of Faith!

Day 20
Unlocking My Optimal Performance

Moment of Truth: Faith is how we unlock optimal performance, spiritually.

Verse to Remember: *"Faith is the confidence that what we hope for will actually happen; it gives us assurance about things we cannot see."*

Hebrews 11:1 (NLT)

Challenge to Implement: *Read Hebrews 11, the Hall of Faith. Then read Hebrews 13:7. Think about who is in your personal Hall of Faith. If they are living, personally thank them for influencing your life in the most profound way.*

Soli Deo Gloria and *Arise!*®

Candice

Day 20 - Unlock Optimal Performance

Candice McField
Arise!® UNIVERSITY
CMU

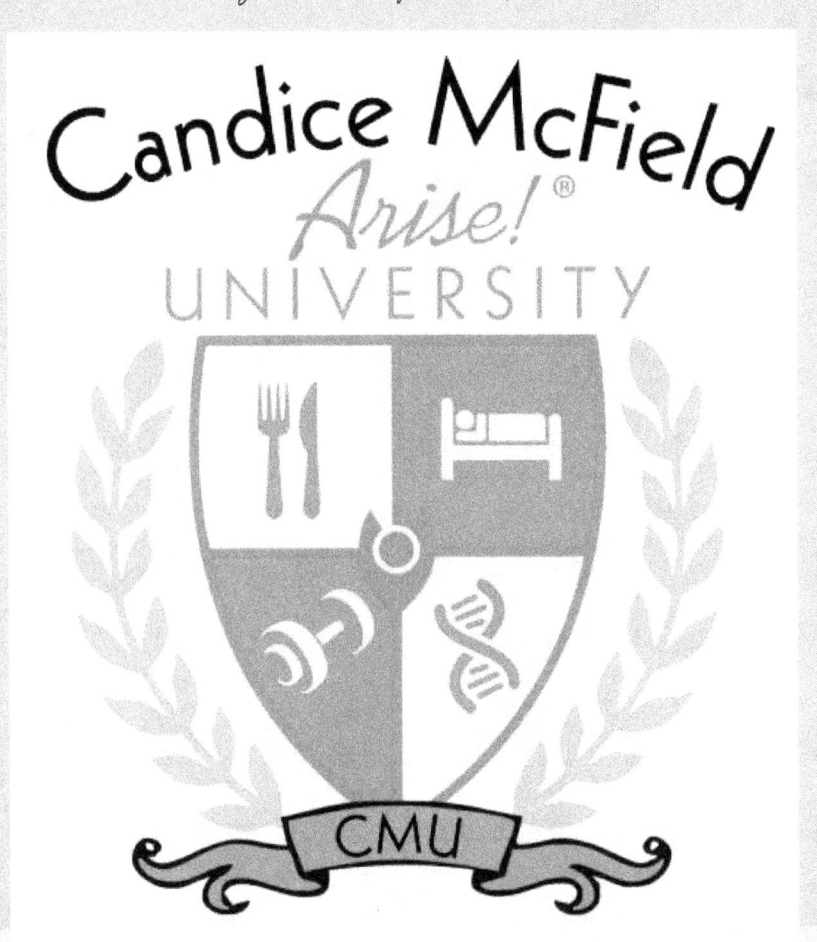

UNLOCK OPTIMAL PERFORMANCE

Understanding your genetics is a key part to physically unlocking your optimal performance. Each of us has certain limitations, which is why we set SMART goals on Day 2. For instance, you may not be equipped to be an Olympic figure skater, win Wimbledon, ever wear a size 2, ever wear a size 22, etc. Genetics play a significant role in your body's composition and its transformation. Unfortunately, most people simply do not have "media body" genes. In fact, most people lack the fortitude and time needed to develop a lean, muscular body with "six pack abs," despite their efforts. It is no wonder why the constant showcase of "Hollywood" physiques cause us to meticulously scrutinize and *be the toughest critics of our own bodies*. Moving forward, I want your primary focus to be unlocking optimal performance for you, and only you!

Because we are all at different stages in our journey, there is only one person in your race to become healthy. Therefore, it is all about you making personal strides and moving forward one step at a time. Sometimes to move forward, we must take a step backwards, or in this case, a look backwards. Knowing and understanding your medical history is very important, including your family's history of diseases, risk factors, and symptoms. A very high percentage of us, have never obtained let alone recorded our family medical history. Knowing you have a predisposition often spurs motivation to unlock optimal performance even greater.

Let's take a look backwards.

Your Medical Information

1. How would you describe your present state of health?
O very well   O healthy   O unhealthy   O ill   O other_____

2. Are you taking any prescription medications?   O yes   O no
If yes, what medications and why?

Do these interact with foods or weight loss in any way?

3. Do you take any over the counter medications or supplements?
O yes   O no
If yes, what medications and why?

4. When was the last time you visited your physician?

5. Have you ever had your cholesterol checked?   O yes   O no
What were the results?   Date of test:

Total Cholesterol: HDL:

LDL: TG:

Your Medical Information Chart from The American Council on Exercise, *ACE Lifestyle & Weight Management Coach*

Day 20 - Unlock Optimal Performance

6. Have you ever had your blood sugar checked? ○ yes   ○ no
What were the results?   Date of test:

---

7. Check all which apply to you and list any important information:

- ○ Allergies
- ○ Amenorrhea
- ○ Anemia
- ○ Anxiety
- ○ Arthritis
- ○ Asthma
- ○ Celiac disease
- ○ Chronic sinuses
- ○ Constipation
- ○ Crohn's disease
- ○ Depression
- ○ Diabetes
- ○ Diarrhea

- ○ Disordered eating
- ○ Intestinal problems
- ○ GERD (gastroesophageal reflux disease)
- ○ High blood pressure
- ○ Hyper-/hypothyroid
- ○ Hypoglycemia
- ○ Insomnia
- ○ Intestinal problems
- ○ IBS (irritable bowel syndrome)
- ○ Irritability
- ○ Menopausal symptoms
- ○ Osteoporosis

- ○ PMS
- ○ Polycystic ovary disease
- ○ Pregnant
- ○ Ulcer
- ○ Skin problems
- ○ Major surgeries:
- ○ Past injuries:
- ○ Any other condition that you may have:

Your Family History

8. Has anyone in your immediate family been diagnosed with any of the following?

○ Heart disease   If yes, what is the relation?
                         Age of diagnosis:

○ High cholesterol   If yes, what is the relation?
                         Age of diagnosis:

○ High blood pressure   If yes, what is the relation?
                         Age of diagnosis:

○ Cancer   If yes, what is the relation?
                         Age of diagnosis:

○ Diabetes   If yes, what is the relation?
                         Age of diagnosis:

○ Osteoporosis   If yes, what is the relation?
                         Age of diagnosis:

After completing the above sections, pick one identified risk area from your medical history and one from your family's medical history to further learn about. How can you prevent, diminish and best of all eliminate any potential risks you may be exposed to?

In the face of new challenges, it is human nature to regress to what is comfortable or seems "normal". Therefore, when new, "abnormal" behaviors appear, you may do fine at first. Yet if these behaviors are not constantly reinforced, you are more likely to revert to your "normal" old habits. Implementing these four paradigm shifts will help you break this pattern.

1. Your new nutritional habits are a lifestyle, not a diet.
2. Regular exercise is your new normal.
3. You value your sleep.
4. You understand your genetic and familial predispositions.

Throughout your health and fitness journey, you will begin to adjust to your "new normal". Remember to unlock optimal performance, exercise is 100% necessary. Nutrition is 100% necessary. Rest is 100% necessary. And Understanding your genetics is 100% necessary. Without all four, reaching the upper limits of performance and body change is nearly impossible! The bullseye, unlocking optimal performance, lies in the intersection of all four.

Day 20 - Unlock Optimal Performance

Day 20
Unlocking My Optimal Performance

Moment of Truth: Understanding your genetics is a key component to unlocking optimal performance, physically.

Quote to Remember: *"Your primary focus is to unlock optimal performance for you, and only you!"*
- Candice McField

Challenge to Implement: Interview your parents regarding their medical history. How can you prevent, reduce, or eliminate any potential risks in which you may be predisposed? Secondly, during the past 20 days you have formed new life changing habits. For each category identify the new habit you are most proud of and/or identify a challenge you will continue to focus on.

Soli Deo Gloria and *Arise!*®

Candice

	Unlock Optimal Performance
Nutrition	The habit I'm most proud of is:
	The challenge I will continue to focus on is:
Strength Training	The habit I'm most proud of is:
	The challenge I will continue to focus on is:
Rest	The habit I'm most proud of is:
	The challenge I will continue to focus on is:
Genetics	The habit I'm most proud of is:
	The challenge I will continue to focus on is:

As For Me and My Body

Relapse Prevention

Identify your goal weight, clothes size, etc. Whatever measurement factor(s) are most important to you. Next, identify your relapse prevention goal weight, clothes size, etc. Ex: If your goal weight is 130 pounds you could set your relapse prevention weight at 135 pounds. Hence, if you get back up to 135 pounds that is your signal to tighten up your workout and nutrition regimen.

Goal 1

Relapse Prevention Goal

Goal 2

Relapse Prevention Goal

Goal 3

Relapse Prevention Goal

Day 20 - Unlock Optimal Performance

Day 21

Arise!® to a New You

For believers, the most significant day in our lives is the day we invite Christ into our lives as our Lord and Savior. The second most significant day is the day we decide to publicly declare our faith in Christ through baptism.

Baptism in the Holy Spirit serves two purposes, an internal and external one. Internally, we immerse ourselves in God, while externally, we clothe ourselves with Him. To be filled inwardly and clothed outwardly with the Holy Spirit is indescribable. There is absolutely nothing like it.

I am thankful to have captured my intimate thoughts regarding my baptism with the following journal entries.

Saturday, July 25, 2009, my journal entry read:

> "Tomorrow I will be baptized and am ready to publicly proclaim my faith in You. The decision wasn't mine last time and now is the perfect time as I am at a new church and truly trying to be active and grow in my faith...Thank you Father as I just started the book of Mark today and was able to read about John the Baptist baptizing others, the meaning behind it and how he had the special privilege and honor to baptize Jesus. Jesus, Jesus, Jesus oh how I

As For Me and My Body

love that name.

Thank you, Lord for bringing me to this point in my spiritual journey. For my earthly father's spiritual influence upon me. For him and I being so close, for him sharing the Left Behind book with me.

Lord - as I am getting baptized tomorrow, I pray that You continue to regenerate my heart. I pray that You convict me in the areas my flesh still continues to sin. I pray that you help make a new me. I pray that You help me step out of my comfort zone by serving you more. Lastly, Father I pray Isaiah 60:1 - that I arise and let my light shine - for Your glory is upon me.

Father - let me and help me to be a shining light to Your Kingdom. I am ready to go to the next level in my walk. I am ready to get baptized and publicly declare my faith that you are my Lord and Savior. Please protect and guide me. Send me Father and I will go.

*Love,
Candi"*

Sunday, July 26, 2009, my journal entry read:

"Today is the second most important day of my life as the first is the day I invited Christ to be my Lord and Savior. But today I was baptized and have officially declared that you are my Lord and Savior for the public...Lord I thank you for this day and for ringing me to this moment in time. I feel - actually, I do not even know how to describe how I feel. Maybe joyous, peaceful, renewed and ready to step out of my comfort zone and continue to mature in my walk with You. Lord I know I will not be perfect but please convict me when I sin and help me to truly seek help and have accountability so that I may become sanctified."

Identification, Power, and Service. These are the three

Day 21 - Arise! to a New You

aspects of the Holy Spirit and His work in our lives. To be filled inwardly with the Holy Spirit marks our identification in Him and gives us the power to overcome sin. Lastly, our most important task once becoming believers is to make disciples through serving Him. When I started Candice McField Fitness, my prayer was to serve Him through providing beneficial services to others, this is still my prayer. My goal is not complete, but I am thankful to be this far in my journey in serving you and ultimately, Him. *(Acts 1:8; Romans 8:2; John 6:63; Galatians 5:25)*

The Candice McField Fitness mantra is *Arise!*® and originates from Isaiah 60:1. *"ARISE, Jerusalem! Let your light shine for all to see. For the glory of the Lord rises to shine on you." Arise!*® simply means to move forward, take immediate action toward the positive, and be accountable. Over the last 21 days, I hope you feel you have had the opportunity to *Arise!*®. My prayer and hope are that you say, "As for me and my body, I will serve the Lord!" I know if you do this, then naturally you will arise to a new you.

In closing, as my grandmother said to me one night, thank you, thank you, thank you! I thank you from the bottom of my heart for allowing me the opportunity to impact your life physically, mentally, emotionally and most importantly, spiritually.

I leave you with two verses from the book of Ephesians:
The call of Ephesians 4:22-24,
> *"Throw off your old sinful nature and your former way of life, which is corrupted by lust and deception. Instead, let the Spirit renew your thoughts and attitudes. Put on your new nature, created to be like God--truly righteous and holy."*

The power of Ephesians 2:10,
> **"For we are God's masterpiece."**

As For Me and My Body

Day 21
Unlocking My Optimal Performance

Moment of Truth: May you forever say, "As for Me and My Body™, I will serve the Lord!"

Verse to Remember: *"For we are God's masterpiece. He has created us anew in Christ Jesus, so we can do the good things he planned for us long ago."*

Ephesians 2:10 (NLT)

Challenge to Implement: *If you have been baptized, mark the date in your calendar and begin celebrating this incredible day of significance annually. If you have not been baptized, and you are a believer, are you ready to profess your faith publicly? If so, contact your church today and inform them of your decision. If you are not a believer, are you ready to invite Jesus into your life? If so, tell Jesus you need him and are ready for Him to be your Lord and Savior. If not, I encourage you to read and study the book of John.*

Soli Deo Gloria and *Arise!*®

Candice

Day 21 - Arise! to a New You

As God's Masterpiece, I Am...

1. A child of God (Romans 8:6)
2. Redeemed from the hand of the enemy (Psalms 107:2)
3. Forgiven (Colossians 1:13 14)
4. Saved by grace through faith (Ephesians 2:8)
5. Justified (Romans 5:1)
6. Sanctified (1 Corinthians 6:11)
7. A new creature (2 Corinthians 5:17)
8. Partaker of His divine nature (2 Peter 1:4)
9. Redeemed from the curse of the law (Galatians 3:13)
10. Delivered from the powers of darkness (Colossians 1:13)
11. Led by the Spirit of God (Romans 8:14)
12. A son of God (Romans 8:14)
13. Kept in safety wherever I go (Psalms 91:11)
14. Getting all my needs met by Jesus (Philippians 4:19)
15. Casting all my cares on Jesus (1 Peter 5:7)
16. Strong in the Lord and in the Power of His might (Ephesians 6:10)
17. Doing all things through Christ who strengthens me (Phil. 4:13)
18. An heir of God and a joint heir with Jesus (Romans 8:17)
19. Heir to the blessings of Abraham (Galatians 3:13-14)
20. Observing and doing the Lord's Commandments (Deut. 28:12-14)
21. Blessed coming in and blessed going out (Deuteronomy 28:6)

22. An heir of eternal life (1 John 5:11-12)
23. Blessed with all spiritual blessings (Ephesians 1:3)
24. Healed by His strips (1 Peter 2:24)
25. Exercising my authority over the enemy (Luke 10:19)
26. Above only and not beneath (Deuteronomy 28:13)
27. More than a conqueror (Romans 8:37)
28. Establishing God's Word here on earth (Matthew 16:19)
29. An overcomer by the blood of the Lamb and the Word of my testimony (Rev. 12:11)
30. Daily overcoming the devil (1 John 4:4)
31. Not moved by what I see (2 Corinthians 4:18)
32. Walking by faith and not by sight (2 Corinthians 5:7)
33. Casting down vain imaginations (2 Corinthians 10: 4-5)
34. Bringing every thought into captivity (2 Corinthians 10:5)
35. Being transformed by renewing my mind (Romans 12:1-2)
36. A laborer together with God (1 Corinthians 3:9)
37. The righteousness of God in Christ (2 Corinthians 5:21)
38. An imitator of Jesus (Ephesians 5:1)
39. The light of the world (Matthew 5:14)
40. Blessing the Lord at all times and continually praising the Lord with my mouth (Psalms 34:1)

Day 21 - Arise! to a New You

Are you sabotaging your fitness goals? Is self-sabotage stopping you from arising to a new you? In fitness, like life, you face many obstacles. None of the obstacles you face will ever prove more challenging than when you face yourself. How many times have you seen your fitness journey through to the end? If you have not, what is stopping you? If you answered "me," you are correct. Most people sabotage their efforts before ever starting. Here are some helpful tips to help you overcome self sabotage and finally achieve your fitness goals.

1. **Reprogram your thinking.** There is a popular saying, "You can't build a positive life from a negative mind." The same is true for fitness. Eliminate limiting beliefs and thoughts. Eliminate the words "I can't" and replace them with "I am." Do not focus on what you may not be able to do. Instead, focus on what you can perform. Some things may be too advanced to perform early on. It is not a matter of "I can't," but rather, "I can't right now." Your perspective is everything when it comes to achieving what you want.

2. **Stop comparing yourself to others.** While it is perfectly normal to aspire to reach a level someone you look up to has already achieved, do not make the mistake of comparing yourself to that individual. Comparing your start to their middle or end is a sure way to derail your fitness goals. Remember, you are not competing against anyone other than yourself. Focus on becoming your best version of you. Maintain a photo journal to see where you started and how far you have come. It is only you versus you.

3. **Manage your outcome expectations.** Be realistic in your expected outcomes. If you have never run a day in your life, do not expect to run a 3K in one week. Fitness, like anything else worthwhile, takes time. Take your large fitness picture and break it into smaller, manageable parts. Rather than attempting to sprint to the finish line, pace yourself for the full length of the race.

4. **Implement the power of 10%.** Research proves that weight loss of only 5-10% of your body weight may diminish health concerns associated with being overweight. Focusing on first-step goals like 5-10% weight loss will help propel you to reach your long-term weight goals and is likely to be sustained over time. Once your first goal has been achieved, focus on maintaining the initial weight loss. Alternatively, you may want to set an interval goal of losing additional weight and have an evaluation period after each interval.

Putting these four tips into practice will yield incredible returns on your health and fitness goals. All change begins with self. To do better, we must commit to being better. Change your mind and you can most certainly change your life.

Welcome to your destination! Welcome to your new you! You have worked hard to overcome obstacles and succeed in achieving your fitness goals. One thing important to your continued success is your perspective. Understand that to maintain the results of your efforts, you must continue to overcome obstacles. There is no such thing as perfection so do not beat yourself up about a slip up here and there. At the same time, do not allow yourself to make excuses. Despite being a professional athlete, even I have times when I am not my best. I do not beat myself up about it. Instead, I acknowledge it and seek to identify what is going on in my life at the time. Afterwards, I immediately get back on track. The key is to always remember *where* you started, *why* you started, and *what* it took for you to accomplish your goals. Renew your motivation constantly and in innovative ways to keep it interesting. In the end, this is a lifestyle and to maintain it, you must be committed to living it.

Day 21 - Arise! to a New You

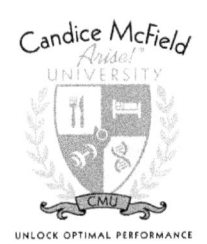

Give a man a fish and he will eat for a day. Teach a man to fish and he will eat for life. CMF teaches fundamentals, hence, clients *Arise!*® and are fit for life!

Arise!®

Over the last 21 days, I have taught you how to fish and not simply eat for the day. I truly believe when you know what to do and understand why you should do it, you are more likely to make wellness a valued part of your lifestyle! I hope you have enjoyed your quest, found it beneficial, and filled with practical, applicable information that you executed and will continue to execute daily.

Finally, I hope it helped you *Arise!*® to a New You!

Candice

As For Me and My Body

Day 21
Unlocking My Optimal Performance

Moment of Truth: Always remember *where* you started, *why* you started, and *what* it took for you to accomplish your goals.

Quote to Remember: "Health and fitness is a lifestyle and in order to maintain it, you must be committed to living it."
— Candice McField

Challenge to Implement: During the past 20 days you have formed new life changing habits. Answer the following questions. Where did you start your fitness quest? Why did you start your fitness quest? Lastly, what did it take for you to accomplish your fitness goals?

Soli Deo Gloria and *Arise!*®

Candice

Arise!® to a New You

Where I started:

Why I started:

What I did to accomplish my goals:

Where I am now:

Author's Reflection

In 2005, I was sitting in a Kingdom Advisors training. The founding director commented how his firm's goal was for clients to gift ten million dollars. I remember sitting and thinking, "Wow, that is it. It isn't about the big house and fancy cars, but joy comes from supporting and giving to things you wholeheartedly believe in." This is the day I added helping others in a significant way to my life goals. It is an objective I did not know where or how to begin achieving until 2010. One day, a thought came to me, to create a fitness solution that strengthens two areas for which I am extremely passionate my relationship with Christ, and keeping my body mentally, physically, and emotionally healthy. It was during my quiet time that I realized, *As for Me and My Body*, would be an incredible way to give to three influential churches in my life.

Your purchase of *As for Me and My Body* has furthered His Kingdom as 10% of the proceeds will be equally distributed to three churches: Koinonia Bible Church, Downtown Church of Christ, and Crossroads Christian Church.

My goal is to sow a significant seed back into Kingdom work. I am confident God will provide as He desires and as He always does. I follow the philosophy of reaching for the

stars because, although you may not reach the star you are striving to reach, you never know what you will accomplish along the way. Regardless of the amount sown into Kingdom work, many lives will be impacted, and three churches will have additional funds for their needs and operation.
Originally written September 8, 2010 (Edited October 28, 2017)

Koinonia Bible Church
The body of Christ I'm honored to call my home church.
    Pastor: Wendell "Deacon" Cole
    7020 Richmond Ave
    Kansas City, MO 64133
    816.313.9130
    koinoniabiblechurch.org

Downtown Church of Christ
My uncle is the head minister of Downtown Church of Christ and a prominent spiritual leader in my life. Hebrews 13:7 says, "Remember your leaders who taught you the Word of God. Think of all the good that has come from their lives and follow the example of their faith." He is a true man of God and an incredible example for all of us to follow.
    Minister: LaVance Anderson
    2010 Van Brunt Blvd
    Kansas City, MO 64127
    816.241.9999
    facebook.com/downtownchurchofchristkc

Crossroads Christian Church
When I started my first health and wellness company, I had nothing but a dream, a business plan, the drive to succeed, and unshakable faith. Crossroads opened their doors to my business partner and me. They allowed us to use their gym facilities without ever asking for anything in return. I am, and will always be, thankful for this blessing.
    Pastor: Brad Fangman
    5855 Renner Road
    Shawnee, KS 66217
    913.962.9966
    crossroadschristian.org

Author's Reflection

As long as Jesus Christ is my Lord and Savior, the sky is the limit as I pour out my heart, remain passionate about my calling, and embrace my full potential. That is what life is all about. I pray that I have influenced your life mentally, physically, emotionally, and most importantly, spiritually. I challenge you to strive for your dreams and reach for the highest star. You never know where you may land along the way. Sixteen years ago, when I worked as a financial research analyst, I never imagined I would be in the position I am today, striving to fight GLOBESITY® internationally. Amazingly, the opportunity is here, and for this, I am thankful. Soli Deo Gloria!

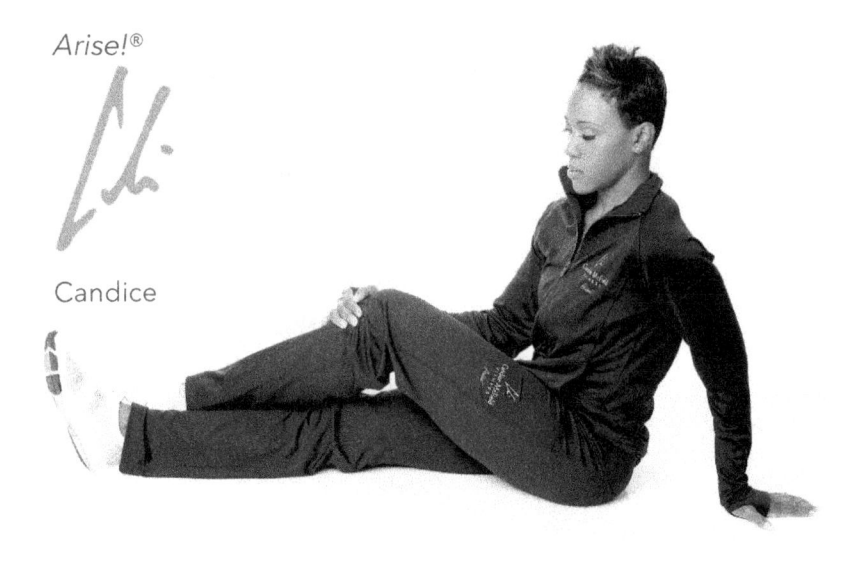

Arise!®

Candice

Acknowledgments

God - For simply allowing me to call you Abba Father.

Mother dear - For instilling the entrepreneur spirit in me and being my number one cheerleader. Most importantly, for providing the love only a mother can give.

Pops - For guiding me back to Christ by giving me the best high school graduation present ever, a bible. One day someone will have some very big shoes to fill as the number one man in my life but regardless, I will always be your Snookums!

Carlos, Sarah, Beckham & Skylar - For giving me an incredible model of the type of loving family I'd be honored to have one day.

Other people I want to thank:
Angelique - For being a trusted sounding board plus always providing calmness and solutions for my panic moments.

Brooke - SB, you are talented beyond belief and CMF would not be where we are without you! Thank you, thank you, thank you!

Cindy - For telling me I need to write this book NOW, not later. Well, "now" is actually years later, but I am so thankful for you nudging me to just do it and for always believing in me.

Collier - For taking my scrambled mumble jumbled thoughts and transforming them into words, sentences, paragraphs, pages, and now a book. You are the hardest worker I know!

Dante - Mi amor, my best friend, and partner in crime for life. Thank you for the joy you add to my life, for loving me unconditionally, and for believing in me.

As For Me and My Body

Frederica - Who would have ever guessed LMU and Gates would lead to a life-long friendship and being family! Thank you so much for all your time and talent to develop the eCourse for this book. You are truly gifted.

Jerry - JC, for believing in me and in CMF with 110% confidence plus for being my partner in crime at Thunderbird! We have had so many incredible times, but I also know the best is yet to come.

LaunchCrate - From little league softball to now a book, we have countless memories and accomplishments that I will always cherish. Creating and publishing this book is the one I am most proud of. Cyndi, thank you for making my dream of becoming an author a reality and for being an incredible publisher!

Sharlie - How can I not love life as our daily jokes and fun help me to always keep things in perspective. Life is too short to not smile and laugh daily. Gracias chica.

Shay - From Phoenix to Denver, to Barbados, many competition trips, photoshoots, businesses, you have been with me every step of the way. I'm just grateful that we both finally decided 'huh she is a pretty cool cousin to have'!

Titia - Our dreams set fire at Semester at Sea, let's keep blazing as no type of dock time will ever hold us down. No words can describe the thanks I owe to you for everything.

Tony - I cannot thank you enough for all your hard work at CMF! You are not only a part of the team, but truly a dear friend!

A special thank you to: My book advisory board Becky, Brooke, Cindy, Darren, Jerry, and LaVance. To team CMF, my family, friends, e23, and clients. To 18 Karat G.O.L.D., Ator, Ayda, Brandy, Chris, Cleve, Crossroads Christian Church, Delta Sigma Theta Sorority, Inc., Delta Sigma Theta Sorority, Inc. Kanas City (KS) Alumnae Chapter, Denny, Downtown Church of Christ, Ethel, Frederica, Gene, Jania, John, Kelly, Keyonna, Koinonia Bible Church, Kristina, Laura, Lisa, Mario, Martin, Pastor A., Ryan, Seth, Stephanie, Susie, and Yesha. Lastly, and to the countless others I've failed to name. Please credit it to my brain and not my heart.

About the Author

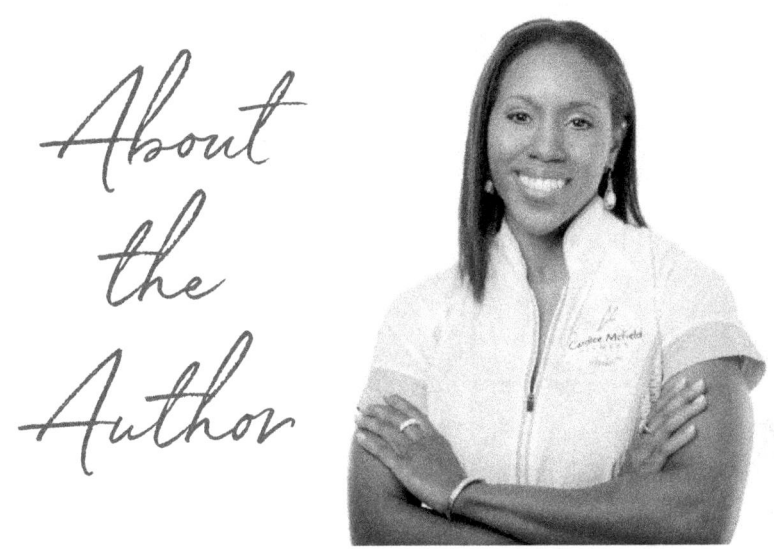

Candice McField is the founder of Candice McField Fitness and As for Me and My Body. She is an ACE Certified Health Coach, fitness educator, and serves on the Kansas Governor's Council on Fitness.

Candice received her Bachelor of Science in Economics from Loyola Marymount University, and an Executive MBA in Global Management from Thunderbird School of Global Management. A natural competitor at a young age, Candice excelled in basketball and softball, but later fell in love with figure competing. Candice's accomplishments include a feature in Oxygen magazines', *Future of Fitness* section, earning her professional card, and securing the 2010 World Natural Bodybuilding Federation "Ms. Figure Universe" title upon her first place finish in Barbados.

Currently, Candice resides in Kansas City where she works with clients internationally and is the host of "Conversations with Candice" on the Fox 4 Kansas City Morning Show.

To learn more about Candice and *As for Me and My Body*, visit: asformeandmybody.com.

Join our Community

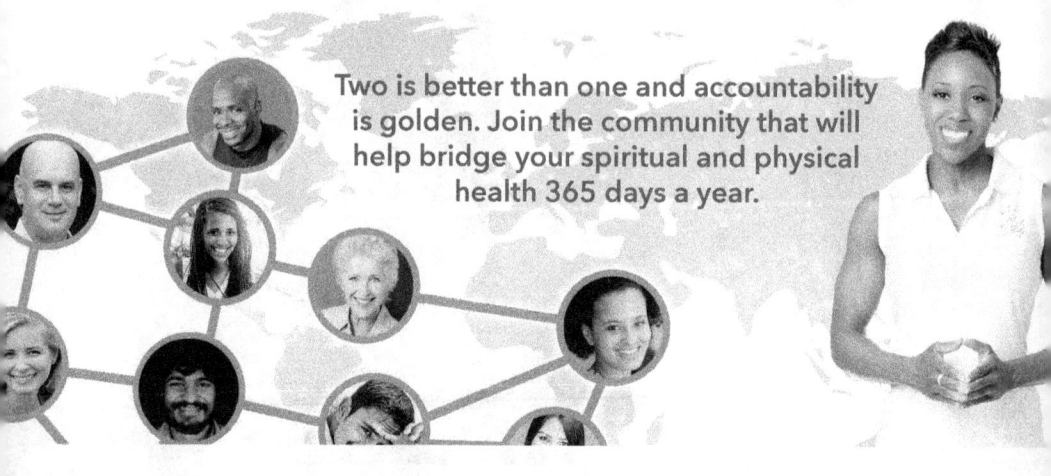

Two is better than one and accountability is golden. Join the community that will help bridge your spiritual and physical health 365 days a year.

To join, go to: asformeandmybody.com

Follow us on Social Media
Facebook: afmamb
Instagram: afmamb
Twitter: afmamb

Personal Notes

As For Me and My Body

Personal Notes

As For Me and My Body

Personal Notes

CPSIA information can be obtained
at www.ICGtesting.com
Printed in the USA
BVHW090050281220
596532BV00014B/183/J